Positive Parenting Solutions 2-in-1 Box Set

Easy Newborn Care Tips + Toddler Discipline Tips - The Official Parents Guide To Raising Your Spirited Child

Author
Lisa Marshall

©Copyright 2019 by Lisa Marshall - All rights reserved.

This book is provided with the sole purpose of providing relevant information on a specific topic for which every reasonable effort has been made to ensure that it is both accurate and reasonable. Nevertheless, by purchasing this book you consent to the fact that the author, as well as the publisher, are in no way experts on the topics contained herein, regardless of any claims as such that may be made within. As such, any suggestions or recommendations that are made within are done so purely for entertainment value. It is recommended that you always consult a professional prior to undertaking any of the advice or techniques discussed within.

This is a legally binding declaration that is considered both valid and fair by both the Committee of Publishers Association and the American Bar Association and should be considered as legally binding within the United States.

The reproduction, transmission, and duplication of any of the content found herein, including any specific or extended information will be done as an illegal act regardless of the end form the information ultimately takes. This includes copied versions of the work both physical, digital and audio unless express consent of the Publisher is provided beforehand. Any additional rights reserved.

Furthermore, the information that can be found within the pages described forthwith shall be considered both accurate and truthful when it comes to the recounting of facts. As such, any use, correct or incorrect, of the provided information will render the Publisher free of responsibility as to the actions taken outside of their direct purview. Regardless, there are zero scenarios where the original author or the Publisher can be deemed liable in any fashion for any damages or hardships that may result from any of the information discussed herein.

Additionally, the information in the following pages is intended only for informational purposes and should thus be thought of as universal. As befitting its nature, it is presented without assurance regarding its prolonged validity or interim quality. Trademarks that are mentioned are done without written consent and can in no way be considered an endorsement from the trademark holder.

YOUR FREE GIFT

with this bundle is double!

Thank you for purchasing this book.

Click on this link to download these FREE tools!!!

http://bit.ly/chidlrencommunicationtips

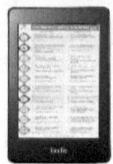

http://bit.ly/childrenbehaviortips

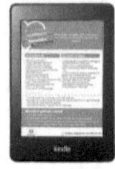

Note: If you have purchased the paperback format then you need to write this link on your browser search bar. These tools are useful resources to:
1. understand the development of the language and communication of children. It is also a checklist for language and listening skills that will provide you with effective tips.
2. understand children's behaviors. It is also a quick guide to connect and respond effectively to your child.

Table of Content

Easy Newborn Care Tips:

Introduction 3
Chapter 1 - Understanding Your Newborn Child's Behavior 8
Chapter 2 - Everything You Need To Know About Breastfeeding Your Child 25
Chapter 3 - Development Of Your Child 79
Chapter 4 - Healthcare For Your Child 103
Chapter 5 - Understanding Sleep Patterns 119
Conclusion 148

Toddler Discipline Tips:

Introduction 161
Chapter 1: Understanding Toddler Behavior 166

Chapter 2: Encouraging Good Toddler Behavior 181

Chapter 3: Behavior Management Tips & Tools 196

Chapter 4: Crying & Tantrums 211

Chapter 5: Common Behavior Concerns 229

Chapter 6: Friends & Siblings 242

Chapter 7: Discipline 255

Chapter 8: Connecting 264

Chapter 9: Toddlers: Communicating 275

Chapter 10: Family Routines 287

Chapter 11: Rules And Consequences 298

Conclusion 314

Easy Newborn Care Tips:

Proven Parenting Tips For Your Newborn's Development, Sleep Solution And Complete Feeding Guide

"The moment a child is born, the mother is also born. She never existed before. The woman existed, but the mother, never. A mother is something absolutely new."
(Osho)

Introduction

Congratulations on downloading *Easy Newborn Care Tips* and thank you for doing so.

There are plenty of books on this subject on the market, thanks again for choosing this one! Every effort was made to ensure it is full of as much useful information as possible, please enjoy it!

The attention and care parents provide to their babies helps them to develop and keeps the baby safe.

The feeling of having a child is beautiful and unique. But it is crucial to know that babies need special care and that care begins right from the moment of their birth.

From the very first day, attention must be paid to dealing with the baby, even to create a bond with both the mother and the father, since this is essential for the development of the child. For you to be prepared with the arrival of your little one, we've crafted this fantastic book that helps you cover up all the essential steps to parenthood and what you need to do to raise your baby well.

While there's a lot that you need to cover up, let's take a look at the five most crucial steps every parent MUST be aware of.

Availability

Your baby needs to be cared for all the time. Care in the beginning, in general, refers to the physical needs of the baby, which includes changing diapers, bathing, and breastfeeding, being wrapped and picked up. Also, your baby is totally dependent on another being to survive, and ideally, the one who can provide this care is the mother. Your baby needs to feel the real presence of his or her mother, as often as possible. In biological children, the attachment of the baby and the mother develop when the baby is in the womb, and the baby will recognize the mother instantly. In adopted newborns, the parents must form and strengthen this bond with their babies. While it's not as easy as it is with biological children, it's possible when you stay available for your baby when they need you.

Routine

For the baby to develop well, it is necessary to have a regular care routine, and the caregiver is the same person, preferably the mother. One day must be equal to the other so that your baby can feel safe. Routine and predictability of care significantly contribute to the baby's ability to organize and develop physically. This routine not only makes it easy for your baby to feel safe, but it also makes it easier for the parents to get stuff done regularly without any surprises.

Sleep

A newborn needs many hours of sleep, which could be anywhere between 15 to 18 hours a day. However, your baby will need to wake up to feed every 2 - 3 hours. The range varies from baby to baby. Some little ones, from birth, sleep through the night, but in most cases, this does not happen. Therefore, it is vital for the mother or father to rest while the baby is asleep so that they are available to take care of the baby when awake. It's not comfortable to sleep for brief intervals so a breast pump can work wonders because the mother can keep bottles handy for the father when it's his turn to hustle with the baby at night.

It is also essential that, from the beginning of the baby's life, a sleep routine is established, so that the baby gets used to it and develops good sleeping habits. Differentiating the day from the night can help your baby to sleep less by day, so it is crucial that you keep the clarity and noises of the house while your baby sleeps during the day, maintain silence and reducing the brightness to the night, as well , so your baby learns to differentiate the day from the night. Over time, this insight helps your baby to sleep more at night.

However, if the baby wakes up, even at dawn, it is important that he or she be attended to. Your baby will wake with any of the following needs, which are usually hunger, pain, or a diaper change. And it's up to the parents to figure out what it is and be available to them, so they grow up to be strong, secure and independent children. Keep reminding yourself that infancy isn't going to last forever and no matter how daunting these tasks seem right now, it's something you will miss most about being a parent.

Holding Your Baby In A Secured Manner

When your baby was in the mother's womb, your baby was wrapped around the walls of her uterus in an aquatic environment, where he or she sensed the balance of his mother's movements, which gave your baby a feeling of warmth. After birth, your baby began to live on a still and rigid surface, which is very different from the maternal womb your baby was accustomed to. Therefore, you need to facilitate the adaptation of this little being and provide a warm cuddle whenever required. A swaddle also works wonders to keep your baby secure while asleep.

It is always the parents who provide security to a newborn. When holding your baby, you need to give him or her as much security and tranquility as possible, so that your baby feels balanced and "safe." The basis of personality will be well-established firmly when your baby is adequately secured. When holding your baby, make sure you have a firm grip over her head, and your other hand is wrapped around your baby's body.

Touching

Touching is critical to the baby's physical and psychological development and is essential for his or her adaptation to the world. Whether it's changing your baby's diapers, bathing, or even a massage routine, the loving touch at any age of the baby contributes significantly to your physical, psychological, and motor development. Some studies show that babies who had their bodies touched and massaged benefited with weight gain, among other benefits related to psychomotor development.

In the early months, it is convenient to leave the baby wrapped in the crib in a blanket with rollers or cushions around them so that he or she can touch them when while moving. This is an excellent way for your baby to feel welcomed, nested, facilitating the adaptation into the world in which you, as new parents have welcomed your bundle of joy!

Now that you've got your basics covered, let's take a closer look at what you need to do to be a hands-on parent to a newborn.

Chapter 1 - Understanding Your Newborn Child's Behavior

Understanding the needs of your child always takes time so you need to be patient once you become a parent. Parenting is a journey and there are going to be hiccups along the way. All you need to do is stay prepared for them and face them together so you can raise a baby that's healthy and happy. You need to remember that all babies are different and while something may have worked really well for one child, it doesn't necessarily mean it will work for your own. You know your baby the best and you will eventually figure out what your child likes and dislikes and what works well for your child. Always speak to a doctor irrespective of what other people tell you. When it comes to taking advice, listen to everybody but do what your heart tells you to do and do not ignore suggestions made from a doctor or a medical representative. The transition from breastfeeding to feeding your baby solid foods is always going to be challenging but as long as you face it with confidence and you give your baby time to adapt, you will manage to feed your baby healthy meals right from infancy till they grow up.

Colic

Although the percentage is very small, babies do develop Colic. Colic is nothing but spells of crying that will last for hours on end. Some babies even end up crying for the entire day or the entire night. There is no medication that is available for colic babies and you need to make sure that you find ways to soothe a baby when this occurs.

How To Prevent Colic While Breastfeeding?

Colic is the condition that causes severe pain in the abdomen of a child and it is usually caused by the kind of food that you eat. Food such as cow's milk, cauliflower, broccoli, and spicy food as well as chocolate can cause colic in a baby. Make sure your baby is healthy and does not suffer from these problems, by avoiding all of these items.

Colic has been a mystery for so many doctors and there are a number of theories related to colic. Colic usually applies to any child that is continuously crying for more than 3 to 4 hours on a daily basis. If this happens for one or two days, then that is absolutely fine. However, if it continues for three or more days in a particular week, then that is a cause for concern. Some children continue crying for more than 3 days a week and this goes on for more than 3 weeks. If you had a full-term baby then colic will usually begin when your baby is around 2 weeks old. If your baby is premature then colic will start later than two weeks. Doctors usually say that colic goes away by the time the baby is 3 or 4 months old. Contrary to belief, the sex of the baby, as well as the feeding habits, does not really affect colic. There is really no difference between people that had colic when they were babies versus people that didn't have colic. Here are a few theories with regards to what may cause colic and how you can help your baby calm down:

- Gas problems
- Hormonal changes that usually result in your baby being in a fussy mood
- The muscles in the digestive system are in pain due to the growth of the digestive system
- Nervous system of your baby slowly developing

Some parents even misunderstand certain conditions like colic and they usually panic. If you are really concerned then make sure that you take your baby to a doctor and find out the reason why he or she may be crying a lot.

Here are a few reasons why your child may be quite irritable and tend to cry a lot:
- An infection that may make your child feel uncomfortable
- Any kind of inflammation in the nervous system or the brain
- A child suffering from irregular heartbeats
- Any minor injury to the muscles or maybe to any of the bones
- Any kind of eye problems that the child may face

Treating Colic
Your doctor will be able to prescribe the ideal treatment for colic based on the tests that are done for your child. Ideally, there are things that need

to be done one step at a time and you will need to see if your child calms down before you try the next step. Before you try too many remedies you should know that colic will get better on its own and you will need to be patient with your baby's development. Here are a few things that you could consider doing in order to ease the discomfort for your baby.

Feeding Habits

Although the feeding habits of the baby are not directly related to colic they can cause a bit of irritation and you need to see if switching between breastfeeding and formula helps reduce the colic in your baby.

Swallowing Air

If your child is facing gas related problems then you could try getting a special bottle that will help him or her swallow less air. You also need to make sure that your child sits up while feeding so that less air goes into the mouth. Also, make it a habit to burp your child during the feeding session and even after the feeding session.

Soothing The Baby

You could try various ways of soothing your baby and calming them down. This could be done with motions such as walking or rocking your child and it could also be done with the help of sounds such as singing for your baby.

Body Language

During the nonverbal stage of a child's development, a child's only way of communicating is through their behavior and body language. Children are very honest and direct and are conveying messages to those around him or her indicating what they need at that time.

By taking the time to watch and listen you will be able to better read the messages that your child is sending you and better respond to and fulfill their needs which will create a happier more well-adjusted child with a greater level of self-esteem. This willingness to read and respond will act positively on the development of the child's personality and temperament. Taking the time to tune in to your child's gestures and nonverbal communication style is essential to their healthy development.

0 - 3 Months

During the first few weeks of life, your newborn seems to send a wide variety of signals. After birth, he turns his head when you touch his cheek, and extends his arms and legs crying when he is frightened, even he takes a step forward when his feet touch a flat surface or grabs your finger when you caress his palm. Dr. Speer (Assistant Professor at Pediatric Surgery at the University of Texas), states that "It is interesting to note that none of these body signals is true communication. These are simply reflexes with which your child was born."

In a few months, some will disappear completely, while others will evolve into more targeted actions. Of course, not all of your baby's first signs are mere reflexes. The smile that emerges at around 6 weeks, for example, is not false. Ron Marino, director of general pediatrics at the Winthrop-University Hospital in Mineola, New York, states that "Your child's smile is not always an answer to your actions, but it is a sign that he is happy... The parents work hard during those first six weeks of the baby's life, and it's nice to have feedback. "

4 - 8 Months

At 4 months of age, your baby's physical signals are clear because he begins to learn the cause and effect and coordinate thought and action. It is and it will be him, from now on, to use signals to indicate his desires and his needs. For example, raising his arms when he wants to be raised or kicks his high chair when he is tired of sitting, or throwing a toy when he wants to play with you because this is a clear invitation to play. Children of this age can also use body language to indicate that playful recreation is over. Signs such as turning himself back or interrupting eye contact usually mean that your child has received enough stimulation or simply wants to play with his toys alone. During this time, our child is able to confuse us with some gestures that do not seem even remotely related to cause and effect. He can, in fact, pull his ears or move his head back and forth to indicate he is tired.

9 - 12 Months

Around 9 months, most children experience an explosion of cognitive growth. Mobility and eye-hand coordination improve, gestures are more specific, clear and communicative. From now on he will be able to easily demonstrate his desires and needs, likes and dislikes. A baby can welcome a familiar face with outstretched hands or cling tightly to the mother or father when anxiety for a stranger begins to emerge.

For example, at 1 year of age, if he is hungry, he can hit the bread drawer in the kitchen, or when he is thirsty, he places himself in front of the refrigerator, but he can also begin to match his signals with a variety of sounds. In a short time, the child's body language will be replaced with simple words and sentences of three words, hoping that they are easy to decipher. That's all? One of the most interesting indicators is the ability to reach intimacy - or links with other human beings - that is directly linked to our first interactions and comfort levels with our parents, primary caregivers.

Mom, I know what you're thinking: "Am I wrong, am I doing something wrong?" Other important ways the baby communicates his needs and desires are shown below. Some may seem obvious, but remember, babies speak an ancient language while adults rely on verbal indicators. Let us then review some linguistic manifestations of the body of our baby.

.

Baby Whining

What should a parent do? Our first communications with people around us are all non-verbal. Have you ever heard a three-day baby ask for a diaper change? No, babies in the first year mostly communicate through body language. And because it can be a source of confusion especially when deprived of sleep - babies cry, contort themselves and make confusion, trying to get proper attention and response, we often misinterpret what they are trying to say.

Getting a firm grasp on what the baby is trying to say allows us to raise that deep, ongoing bond between parent/caregiver and child. For some mothers this bond is immediate, for others it takes time, patience and a bit of work. By paying attention to the newborn's body language, you help facilitate this bond much more quickly - thereby developing the level of intimacy with your baby that needs to feel safe and loved. By understanding a lot of what babies are trying to communicate to us, we are aware that these movements are instinctual, they are the result of eons of evolution. Human beings are born with the ability to communicate - but not with the capabilities of spoken language. The language is artificial, a sub-product of the human condition, born from progress and necessity, not incorporated into our DNA.

For example, the "Moro reflex", common in newborns, is a phenomenon that disappears from the baby's repertoire at the age of four months when they adapt to life outside the womb. When this reflex is solicited, the baby grabs the air with the palms up and the thumbs flexed out and often the legs are similarly positioned. When we see these positions/movements, the child is reacting to fear. This reflex, which usually disappears after 3 or 4 months, is often a response to a sudden loss of support, often when a newborn feels like he is falling. It is normal, but the alarm-wake reflex can be avoided when he's going to sleep.

Head Rolling

The baby turns his head the other way when it is bored, disinterested or overstimulated. It's time to change gear! He rubs his eyes: often accompanied by one or two large yawns, it indicates fatigue. Studies have shown that the act of rubbing the eyes has a calming effect on the heart rate. He pulls and rubs the ears: when a part of our body touches another part, for example, rubbing the chin, screwing the hair, we want to indicate that we need comfort. In an attempt to console themselves, to get ready to sleep or to disengage from a particular situation, babies rub their ears to calm their emotions. It is easier to recognize these movements and gestures than to interpret their meaning. All babies are different, it is important to know and understand their behaviors and effectively establish their cause.

Arched Back

This is an act of rebellion, but when it is over-extended it can be a reaction to pain, almost always to heartburn, the most likely cause. If the newborn arches his back while feeding and crying or spitting excessively, it may be a sign of reflux or gastroesophageal reflux disease, a condition in which acid reflux from the stomach irritates the esophagus. If this behavior does not seem to be linked to nutrition, it can mean frustration and he asks for comfort.

Kicks Continuously

If he looks happy and smiling, this is probably a sign he wants to play, while if he is demanding or crying, it is an indication that something is probably worrying the baby. The cause can be anything from gas colic to a dirty diaper while sitting in a cramped car seat, but they can kick their legs simply because they can.

Head Banging

If you see your 10-month-old baby banging his head, like a wand, methodically on the hardwood floor or against the bars of his crib is an alarming attitude. But many babies do it regularly, and it seems that this does not cause any kind of pain, on the contrary: babies find the rhythmic movement forward and backward soothing. However, it should not be underestimated, up to 3 years, because if the child bangs his head for long periods of time, instead of engaging with others or playing with his toys, the pediatrician should be contacted.

Clenched Fists

Most newborns hold their hands in this resting position because they are not yet able to do much more since the movement of the finger and hand requires a more developed nervous system and more complex brain function. Babies usually start to open their hands at 8 weeks and start reaching and grabbing for 3 or 4 months. Many times clenched fists can be a sign of stress or even hunger. If the baby's tendency to squeeze his fists persists after 3 months, it is good to have a pediatrician visit him.

Bent Knees (On The Abdomen)

This position is usually a sign of abdominal discomfort, or the presence of gas, a bowel movement, or constipation. It is important to try to alleviate the "ahi ahi!" If gas seems to be the problem, help him burp during feeding. If you breastfeed, check your guilty diet for producing gas from broccoli or potatoes. If you think constipation is a problem, it can usually occur when babies switch from breast milk to formula or when they start to taste solid foods around 6 months, check with your pediatrician for nutrition.

Self-Soothing

A number of parents witness their children banging their heads, rocking their body and rolling their heads from side to side at times. While this may seem disturbing to you, be rest assured it is absolutely normal for your child to behave in this manner. The reason they do this is that it helps them to feel comforted and it is part of self-soothing. The common symptoms of self-soothing include:

- Staying in that position and rocking the body back and forth
- Sitting on the bed and banging the head towards the headboard
- Lying face down and banging the head and chest on the pillows or the mattress
- Moving the head from side to side while lying on the back

Making Noises While Rocking
Body rocking can start around 6 months while headbanging and head rolling is something that your child learns by the time they reach the age of 1. This behavior could continue between the age of 1 and 5 years but in some scenarios, children tend to continue the habit even post the age of 5.

Tips To Handle This Behavior
Keep a track of how long your child takes to fall asleep. If you notice that the time span is relatively long then this could cause headbanging in a child. Although a lot of parents want to go and try to control the behavior it is something that you need to stop yourself from doing. Children try to look at this as a method to grab attention and when you begin to notice or tell them to stop this habit will continue to grow.

The best thing to do is to protect your child and ensure that your child will not hurt themselves in any way. Try to get smooth rounded corners in all spaces of the bedroom and keep sharp edges away from your child.

When Do You Need To Seek Help?
While it is normal for a child to put themselves to sleep, if you notice that they do this throughout the night then this may be a concern and you may want to go check with your doctor. Some children

tend to bang their head because of obstructive sleep apnea and it is important for you to treat this condition if you want them to stop.

Some children may suffer from intense conditions and this is why they bang their head and this could include developmental delays, spectrum disorder, autism or blindness. You will be able to differentiate between these habits and the normal headbanging habits if you notice that your child tends to rock the body and bang their head even during the day. While head banging and body rocking are normal when a child is trying to sleep, if your child is doing it even while they are awake then this is something you need to pay attention to.

Decoding Baby Crying

When the baby cries, he can have very different needs. We must not be taken immediately by anxiety and the fear that he is suffering, but concentrate on the characteristics of crying, listening to him, observing the baby's behavior to try to interpret his signal and respond appropriately. Here is a guide to help you evaluate the various nuances of the baby's crying.

I'm Hungry!

"Hunger cries usually begin as a low-intensity whine, then progressively increases, if the baby's need is not met, at the acute screams," explains

Andrea Dotta, Director of the Neonatal Intensive Care Unit of the Bambino Gesù Pediatric Hospital in Rome. "It stops immediately when the baby is offered the breast, while the pacifier can only calm it for a few moments. To understand if a child is crying from hunger, of course, it is good to remember when he was fed last time, how long he sucked and if he sucked enough milk. "

Colic, Reflux And...
Immediately begins with shrill cries. "It's not a whine, but a scream," says the neonatologist. "In this way, the evening crying crises of babies suffering from colic or those of the little ones who have gastroesophageal reflux usually begin. Sometimes the crying of suffering can temporarily subside if the baby is offered the pacifier or, even better, the breast because the movement of suction stimulates the release of endorphins and reduces pain. We must therefore be careful to not confuse it with the cry of hunger. The baby who suffers can suck for a while, but then it comes off and inevitably starts to cry again ". The most frequent causes in newborns are gaseous colic, gastroesophageal reflux, and otitis.

"The baby is not able to describe his disorder, but parents can get some clues from his attitude and his movements. "If crying occurs with a certain regularity every day or almost, in the late afternoon or evening and the baby tends to contract the legs and flex them on the tummy, it is probably gaseous colic. There are no definitive remedies to eliminate the pain of colic, but usually, those babies who suffer from it benefit greatly from the tummy massages and from standing on their stomach, possibly in a belly-to-belly contact with their mother ".

The reflux tears occur instead during and after meals, because of the pain that the baby feels is due to the ascent of the gastric contents, which irritates the mucous membrane of the esophagus. "The baby breaks away from the breast frequently, bends his head back and arches his back," says the expert. Finally, otitis is more common in babies who are already a few months old than newborns. "Mom and Dad can recognize it by touching the baby's ears and watching his reaction," says Dotta. "In case of suspected reflux or otitis, it is necessary to consult the pediatrician for the diagnosis and appropriate treatment".

Discomfort
It is a less intensity lamentation than the cry of pain. "It is a sign that there is a discomfort factor in the environment where the child is: too much noise, too much light, too hot or cold, or a wet diaper," explains the expert. "Usually, the crying of the newborn has a plaintive cadence, without screams or sharp peaks, but it can grow in intensity if the cause of the problem is not removed."

Cuddles Time?

Does it make sense for a baby to talk about crying for a tantrum? "I would say no, at least not in the meaning that we attribute to this word for older children: sometimes, the little one cries because he wants to attract the attention of parents", Dotta replies. "He gets bored and wants to interact with adults and the environment, seeking the gratification of a mother's embrace and cuddles". Understanding the reason for crying of a newborn is easy: to calm him, it is enough for the mother to take him in her arms, talk to him and keep him close to her. It is important to satisfy the need for physical contact of the newborn. For nine months, in maternal uterus, he experienced a condition of containment and, after birth, he needs to relive it in the embrace, in the skin-to-skin contact with the mother, in the rocking movement of her walk while cradling him, in the caresses. They are indispensable gestures to create the bond of attachment between mother and baby, and for the healthy, harmonious development of the future personality of the child.

Chapter 2 - Everything You Need To Know About Breastfeeding Your Child

Understanding Breastfeeding

Breastfeeding is something every woman should experience after childbirth not only because it helps to emotionally connect with the child but also because it has a lot of health benefits for the mother as well.

Breastfeeding Benefits For Mothers

Breastfeeding is healthy for women and there are a number of reasons why women should not shy away from providing their child with breast milk for at least 6 months. When a woman breastfeeds a child, it helps her to connect with her child, making her feel happy as a person. Women who breastfeed are less likely to suffer from postpartum depression and tend to be happier. They also look forward to nurturing the child and connecting with the child more effectively. This is because breastfeeding releases good hormones that help take out the physical and emotional drain that a woman experiences during pregnancy. It releases two main hormones which include:

• Prolactin - This hormone helps to enhance the nurturing sensation in a woman and relaxes the child which focuses on the development during the early stages of infancy.

• Oxytocin - Helps build a strong bond between the mother and the child and makes a mother feel happy to hold the child close to her.

Women who breastfeed their baby post-childbirth manage to recover from pregnancy-related problems faster. Regular feeding helps to reduce the size of the uterus and bring it back to pre-pregnancy size a lot faster. It also helps to reduce postpartum bleeding which could drain a lot of energy out of a woman.

Women who breastfeed are less likely to suffer from ovarian cancer and they also manage to lose pregnancy weight more effectively in the process. It also helps women to reduce the risk of suffering from type 2 diabetes, cardiovascular disease, high blood pressure and high cholesterol and rheumatoid arthritis. Exclusive breastfeeding also acts as a contraceptive (Lactational Amenorrhea Method or LAM) because it helps to delay the menstrual cycle of a woman. This helps the body to cope with one pregnancy at a time and ensures that the second pregnancy does not occur too quickly. Breastfeeding caters to a motherly instinct in a woman that helps fulfill the urge to become a mother. It is also convenient because the mother doesn't have to worry about packing up too many things while traveling with a small baby. Breastfeeding is an affordable solution in comparison to the formula that could cost you a lot of money.

Breastfeeding Benefits For Babies

There is no denying that breast milk is the best food for your baby and the advantages that this kind of milk offers are aplenty. Doctors all across the world encourage new mothers to breastfeed for as long as possible because it is natural and an integral part of the development of your baby. Even if you can breastfeed your child for as long as six months, it is something you definitely need to consider doing.

Breast milk contains a number of live ingredients which include healthy bacteria, stem cells, white blood cells, antibodies hormones and enzymes that work together to fight infections and prevent a number of diseases that occur in babies who are not breastfed. Babies who are breastfed are more likely to develop and grow healthier as compared to those who are not because they miss out on a lot of vital nutrients during the first stage of life. Breastfeeding decreases the chances of diarrhea or gastrointestinal infection as well. It is also less likely that a child who is breastfed suffers from an ear infection or chest infection from time to time.

The rate of sudden death infant syndrome in babies is higher when they are fed formula milk. Let's not forget the main reason why it is important to breastfeed your child. It is because it soothes a crying baby much like it provides comfort to someone who is hurt, and most parents underestimate how essential this is for the development of their baby.

Breastfeeding Premature Babies

Premature babies are more prone to conditions such as infections as well as fatal life-threatening diseases like chronic lung disease or sepsis. Nursing a premature baby with mother's milk can reduce the risks and can also increase the likelihood of the baby going home a lot sooner. Premature babies who are not provided with breast milk take a longer time to develop and become healthy in comparison to the babies who are nursed on a regular basis.

Help Babies Sleep Better

Breastfeeding enhances the sleep quality of a child and also enables a baby to go back to sleep faster as compared to when fed with formula. The more regular your baby's sleep and wake patterns are, the healthier your baby will grow and the faster you will notice development signs in a child.

Brain Development

The first six months are crucial in the development of a baby because this helps the growth of the brain increase at the speed that will never occur through the rest of the baby's life. If you want your baby's brain to develop in a healthy way, it is best to breastfeed. Children that feed through breastfeeding are more likely to achieve the desired milestones during the first six months in comparison to a baby that is fed formula milk. These children also tend to come out smarter and have higher IQs. The fatty acid present in milk is what enhances brain development and create a positive effect on the child. These fatty acids are only found in breast milk and cannot be replicated through any other formula.

It is also believed that babies that are breastfeeding do not suffer from behavioral issues as compared to children who are not. Children who are bottle-fed turn out to be more stubborn than the ones who were on breast milk for the first six months of their life. Even when you transcend to feed your baby healthy food, try to limit the use of the bottle as much as possible.

The benefits of breastfeeding are not just for the first six months of your baby but for a lifetime. Children develop a sense of security and attachment with their families and this helps them to deal with stress more effectively even when they grow up. Breastfed babies are less likely to suffer from various kinds of cancer such as lymphoma and leukemia. These babies also have better eyesight and stronger teeth. Breastfed babies are less likely to gain too much weight and become obese or suffer from diabetes. Let's not forget, breastfeeding is an economical way to nurture and nourish your baby in the healthiest possible manner.

Benefits Of Breastfeeding On Families

There is no denying that breastfeeding provides numerous benefits to the mother. It helps them develop a strong bond and keep them both healthy. Apart from being a great source of nutrition to the child, there are various other benefits of breast milk that can work well for the entire family.

No Expensive Equipment Or Formula Required

One of the major benefits of breastfeeding your baby is that you will be able to do so even in an economic environment without having to worry about spending too much money. Infant formula costs a lot of money and apart from investing in the formula; one also needs to take into consideration the tools and accessories required to prepare formula in a healthy manner. All of these items cost a lot of money and when a woman breastfeeds, she can eliminate these costs, making it easy for the family to cope with the additional member gradually.

Less Medical Expenses

There is no denying that babies who depend on formula fall ill more often and are prone to infection, including bottle infection that happens due to improper sterilization of the bottle or the other equipment used in the process. Children who are not breastfed also need to depend on various other medications to help them develop and this costs more money.

Emotional Stability

Babies who are not breastfed tend to get more insecure as they grow. Breastfeeding creates a natural bond between the mother and child and when this stage is eliminated, it becomes difficult for the child to adjust in a new environment. Babies who are not breastfed tend to get crankier as they grow and it becomes more difficult to handle them.

It Works As A Contraceptive

Research has shown that a woman who breastfeeds her child is less likely to get pregnant again in the first few months after childbirth (also known as Lactational Amenorrhea). This helps her body adjust to the new changes and still manages to keep her life normal with her family.

Time-Saving

A woman does not have to worry about the time that is required to prepare a meal for the babies because breast milk is always available. Infants are required to be fed multiple times a day and when a woman can breastfeed, it makes it easy for her to attend to the baby a lot faster and soothe the baby more effectively.

Less Stressful

A new mother is constantly worried about how she is going to look after her baby and when she has to think about an external factor of preparing formula, it puts more stress on her. Regular breastfeeding reduces the stress of having to worry about constantly being ready with food and always worrying about whether or not it will run out. It allows a woman to move around with her baby more confidently, knowing for a fact that she will be able to feed the hungry baby irrespective of where they are.

Tips For Your First Breastfeeding Experiences

The first 24 hours of a woman who is giving birth is more of what we could call a roller coaster ride. There's a lot of emotions and stress that women go through and it's also a crucial stage for her to begin the journey of breastfeeding her baby. There are a lot of questions in the mind of a woman when they first begin to breastfeed. Here is a complete guide that will help you understand exactly what you need to do to breastfeed your child during the first few days post-birth.

Start Early

The sooner you begin breastfeeding, the more comfortable you will get with the concept and the healthier it will be for your baby. You should start feeding your baby the minute you get to hold your baby for the first time. Ideally, you should nurse the baby for at least an hour once you give birth so that your baby gets used to you as soon as possible and you have no trouble in feeding the child. If you cannot feed your baby immediately after birth, you may want to consider purchasing a breast pump to assist you. If your breast doesn't naturally secrete enough milk, then the best thing for you to do would be to use a breast pump because this will considerably increase the amount of milk that is produced and it will help you to feed your baby conveniently.

Check For An Early Latch

A baby latches onto the mother almost instantly and it figures out a way to circle the nipple even when they are just a few hours old. If your baby has not latched on in the first few attempts, then you may have a latching on issue. This is, however, a very rare scenario where babies do not manage to latch on to their mothers independently.

Babies Sleep Deep

Once the baby is born, they often fall into a deep sleep after a few hours and will not be able to latch as effectively as they could just after they were born. In certain cases, the baby latches on to you faster and they learn how to suck milk out of your breast and it makes the process of feeding the baby that much easier. Even if you haven't managed to get hold of a breast pump almost instantly and your baby wasn't able to drink milk soon after birth, there is no need for you to stress. You can always try and breastfeed a little later.

Breastfeeding - Days 1 To 3

Nurse Frequently

For the first few days post-delivery, you should keep your baby as close as possible because you will not be able to understand the exact feeding schedule of your child. When in the hospital, try to keep your baby skin to skin as much as possible so that you understand exactly when your baby is looking for the breast and you'll be able to feed your baby at the right time. Head bobbing, fist sucking and mouth fluttering are early signs of hunger, and this will let you know that you have to feed your baby.

No Artificial Nipples

You may not be able to nurse your baby very often but that doesn't mean that you should provide your baby with an artificial nipple or a pacifier to stay calm. A baby's stomach is small and all the milk that your baby needs is being produced by you. Avoid these pacifiers for as long as possible.

Colostrums Are Essential

For the first three days you lactate, your body produces a kind of milk known as colostrums. This milk is not a lot in quantity but it is the richest form of food your baby can get because it contains the necessary vitamins, proteins, antiviral agents and antibodies that help your baby get strong. This is the milk that works as a laxative for your baby and helps them poop.

Weight Loss

During the first three days of nursing, it is normal for your baby to lose about 7% of their weight. This is mainly because of the fact that they start pooping and the other fluids that were accumulated in their body start getting out of the system naturally. Most mothers believe that their baby is losing weight because they are not able to provide enough milk for the baby. The truth, however, is that your baby's stomach is the size of a marble and it eats no more than the amount that your body is producing. Switching to formula at an early stage may complicate matters for your baby and it may not work as well on your baby's digestive system.

Latching On Issues

If your baby hasn't latched on to you yet, there is no need for you to stress during the first few days; but if you are unable to nurse your child at all, then you may want to seek the advice of a doctor. There are going to be a lot of people who will come forward to give you unsolicited advice even though they have no medical background. The best thing for you to do is to avoid these and wait for the doctor and see what they have to say. You should also ensure you keep your baby skin to skin for as long as possible because some babies may find it a little difficult to latch on immediately but they may eventually. In the meanwhile, you should also extract the milk from your breast with the help of a pump and feed it to your baby with a dropper or a small spoon.

Breastfeeding - Days 3 To 5

Your body should get adjusted to breastfeeding during this time and it gets easier for you to understand the schedule of your baby.

Better Milk Flow

By the third to the fifth day, the amount of milk your body produces increases tremendously and you become more accustomed to feeding your baby. Children also learn how to suckle faster and they learn how to drink more milk. It is during this time that you will notice your breasts growing thicker and fuller and if you are using a pump, you will also manage to measure the amount of milk that your body produces.

Overfilling Is Normal

Some babies may not drink as much milk as others and it may be difficult for them to latch on as effectively as well. If your baby is not latching on, the best way to prevent overfilling is to use a breast pump. Some babies have a strong appetite and in this situation, you will not need to worry about your breast overfilling because they will constantly drain out the milk by drinking it at regular intervals.

Hand Expressing

Sometimes your breasts get so full of milk that it is difficult for your nipples to come out and this makes it very inconvenient for the baby to suckle. In such situations, you can use reverse pressure by using softening techniques to help the nipple enter the mouth of your child. Hand expressing is basically holding the nipple between two fingers and trying to drain out a little milk to help your baby.

Gently Massage

Sometimes your breasts become so full with milk that it becomes difficult for the milk to come out conveniently and in such situations, massages can work wonders. Using an ice pack in between the feeding session can help relieve the soreness in the breast and also helps with the flow of milk.

Check Diapers

As soon as you start breastfeeding your baby, you will notice that the color of your baby's poop changes from a greenish-brown color to a light mustard yellow. You will also notice the frequency of the diapers getting wet will increase.

Breastfeeding - Days 5 To 7

By the time you reach the fifth day of nursing your child, you would have gotten accustomed to the routine of your child as well as how long you need to breastfeed your baby. Babies do not like to drink a lot of milk at one time but they need you almost every 2 hours which means you will be breastfeeding your child at least 10 times in a span of 24 hours.

Understanding Your Baby's Hunger

Once the milk starts flowing effectively, you will notice an increase in the weight of your baby. You may want to try and increase the time frequencies in between feeding your child but the minute you notice the signs of hunger such as fist sucking or head bobbing, remember that these are signs that your baby wants milk.

Feeding Time Can Change

Some babies have a fixed schedule with regards to when they need to be nursed and when they need to be put down to sleep, while there are others who do not. Sometimes they decide they are hungry even after they have just got a stomach full of milk. This is normal and it just shows that your baby is also learning to adjust to a routine.

Continue Checking Diapers

A healthy infant will poop at least three to five times in a span of 24 hours. It is important that there is enough quantity of poop and it should be in yellowish in color and sometimes seedy in texture. The color of the poop can also vary depending on what you have eaten. While some babies poop immediately after every feed, there are others who like to consolidate their poop and let it go in one shot. Usually at least 5 to 6 wet diapers are considered normal.

Check Your Baby's Weight

It is important for you to check your baby's weight as often as possible with a digital weighing scale since this is most reliable. In taking the right weight of your baby, try to keep your baby on the weighing machine without any clothes each time.

Get Help If Needed

It takes about two weeks for babies to go back to their original birth weight but by the end of the first week, you will notice a slight change in the weight. If your baby hasn't gained any weight after a week, consider visiting a doctor.

Take Supplements

Women usually focus on a lot of prenatal supplements while they are expecting but they tend to forget taking care of themselves once the baby comes along. If you want your baby to stay healthy, you need to stay healthy as well because at the end of the day your baby gets their nutrients from you. Not all mothers may be required to take supplements but always ask your doctor if you need any.

Tenderness Should Subside

By the fifth to the seventh day, nothing should be uncomfortable for you and you will not experience any pain when your baby is suckling. If it continues paining, then you need to visit a doctor. When your baby first latches on, there will be some mild tenderness that should fade away almost instantly but if it continues for more than a few weeks, then there is a problem and a doctor should definitely be consulted.

Once you pass the first week of breastfeeding, it becomes comfortable for you to feed your child whenever the baby is hungry and you will also be able to figure out exactly what your baby needs and when. Your body becomes accustomed to breastfeeding and you learn the most comfortable position in which you can feed your baby most effectively. This is also the state you should learn to start snuggling with your baby and increase the emotional equation.

Answers To Common Questions About Breastfeeding

There are a number of questions that come to mind for a new mother when she begins breastfeeding. Here we will try to cover as many of them as possible so that you have answers to all your questions when you embark on your journey of nourishing and nurturing your baby.

When Will Milk Start To Form?

Most pregnant women worry about milk not accumulating in their breast during the first few days of their pregnancy. The truth is your body has already started to produce a thick milky substance called colostrums which begins to form before childbirth and will be available in your breast for at least three days post-birth. The milk in your body will start to form after about two or three days and the quantities will continue to increase as you feed your baby.

Does The Size Of The Breast Affect The Amount Of Milk?

It is common for women with smaller breasts to worry about whether or not they will be able to feed their baby and produce enough milk. However, you need to understand that the size of your breast has nothing to do with the amount of milk that your body can produce because this depends on the mammary glands. And as soon as your baby drinks milk, your body will start producing more milk.

Why Is My Baby Still Hungry After A Feed?

While this is rare, sometimes you may not be able to produce enough milk to feed your baby. If the milk supply in your body is low, you can always speak to a doctor or an expert to help increase the production of milk.

Is Breastfeeding Easy?

This is the toughest question to answer because while breastfeeding is the most natural thing to do, it's not the easiest thing for every woman to begin in the first place. The initial few days are a struggle and usually accompanied by a lot of discomfort and pain but once women get past this stage, they will manage to nurse their baby more effectively and without any discomfort.

I Can't Tell If My Baby Is Drinking?

Sometimes a baby immediately latches onto your nipple but may not suck the breast. Sometimes they circle without drinking milk at all and this often confuses you with regards to whether or not your baby has a full stomach. You may want to see whether your breast feels lighter after feeding and this will help you determine whether your baby drank milk or whether your baby was just seeking comfort.

Is My Body Producing Enough Milk?

If your baby seems to be satisfied after a feed and stays relaxed for about 2 or 3 hours post-feed, there is nothing that you should worry about. Post-feed, babies take a good nap and relax, and this is a sign of a full stomach. You will also notice the difference between your breast before and after nursing. With the change in your baby every week, it is also a great way to observe whether you are giving your baby enough food or not.

How To Increase The Milk Supply?

There are a number of reasons why there is less milk produced in your body and if you think that the only way to increase the production of milk includes feeding your baby more frequently, you should know that pumping your breast soon after your baby has been fed and eating a healthy diet and drinking fluids also help. You also need to make sure you get enough rest so that you give your body the time to produce milk.

Soothing The Breast?

It is common for women to experience soreness in the breast and pain during the first few attempts at breastfeeding. Using a breast pump to release the milk or even an ice pack can help you to handle the pain.

How To Cure Sore Nipples?

Sore nipples are common during breastfeeding which is why you need to ensure that you do your best to prevent this condition and treat it as soon as possible. The minute your nipple starts to feel a little sensitive after feeding, try to dry them instead of immediately covering it up with clothes. Do not wear tight-fitting bras or clothes that can stick to your nipple because this can irritate the skin and cause a lot of soreness. Rubbing your nipple with a little breast milk is also a great way to help heal them.

Nursing If My Nipples Are Bleeding?

A lot of women tend to stop breastfeeding when the nipple starts to bleed. Apart from this being uncomfortable, they also believe that it could cause harm to the baby. The truth is that a little blood in your milk will not harm your baby in any way as long as you are healthy and you do not have any contagious illness. While cracked nipples or bleeding nipples do not occur so often, it usually happens when a baby has not latched onto the breast properly.

What To Eat Or Drink While Breastfeeding?

The one thing you need to keep in mind during breastfeeding is that moderation is essential. Well balanced and wholesome diets are something that will help you to provide the night nutrition to your baby and keep you healthy as well. Try to stay away from food items that will make you feel bloated. Drink a lot of water and consume fresh fruits as much as possible.

Is Breast Pumping Healthy?

Breast pumping is extremely beneficial to women who are not able to nurse the child naturally or whose baby has had a problem latching on almost instantly. It also comes in handy when a woman needs to go back to work and cannot stay home for the full day to breastfeed her baby. As long as the breast milk is stored nicely, it can be used to feed a baby later.

How Long Should You Breastfeed?

Some women prefer breastfeeding for up to as long as four years but this isn't something you should do if your baby has started to eat healthy food. Breastfeeding your child for the first six months without the introduction of any other food is necessary. Post 6 months, you should try and introduce your baby to solid foods so that your child learns to become more independent.

Getting Accustomed To Breastfeeding

Once you get past the first few weeks of breastfeeding, it will all be about learning how to accustom yourself to techniques that work well for you. Different women learn to adjust to breastfeeding with different methods. So you need to see what you are most comfortable doing and how well your baby is adjusting to breastfeeding so that you can benefit from it the most.

There are some suggestions that are great for breastfeeding while there are others that should be avoided. If you are not too sure whether you have found the right position to breastfeed your baby, then here are some positions that may help you.

The Cross Cradle Hold

One of the best positions to nurse your child is the cross-cradle position. For you to nurse your baby effectively in this position, you need to be in an upright sitting position on a chair or a sofa that has an armrest. Bring your baby to your front and cross your arms as if you are cradling your baby around the body. Make sure your baby is as close to you as possible before you begin nursing. Your arms should be across from one another which means your left arm should control your right breast while the right arm should support the left. In case you do not have a chair or a sofa with an armrest, you can always use pillows as support. It is important for you to gently guide your baby towards your breast without leaning over your child.

When breastfeeding, keep in mind that it is important for your baby to breathe so the more you try to push yourself on your baby, the more the chances of suffocation. In babies who have difficulty to latch on the breast, it becomes easier for them to use this method because you will be able to guide your baby's head with your hand. Children also feel secure in this position because they are wrapped around in their mother's arm. You can also use this position to feed your baby while sitting on a bed by simply crossing your legs for support.

The Cradle Hold

If you are not comfortable with the cross-cradle position, you can try the cradle position which is very similar to cross-cradle, except that you will not be crossing your arms from one another but rather using your elbow as support. Different women have different body structures so it becomes difficult for them to use a cross-cradle without putting too much pressure on the baby. If you do not want to stretch your baby out, then keep a pillow on your lap and use the cradle position to begin nursing. In the cradle position, you can use your elbow as a guide to help take your baby's head towards the nipple. When nursing your baby in a cradle position, make sure that your baby is straight and not turned to the side because this could cause suffocation during nursing.

The Football Hold

When you have a natural childbirth, it becomes easier for you to begin breastfeeding since there are no stitches on your stomach and you heal faster. However, in the case of a c-section, women take longer to heal and they find it difficult to breastfeed with a baby on the lap. If you have had a C-section and you cannot use the cradle or the cross-cradle position to feed your baby, you can try the football hold. This is convenient since it doesn't put any pressure on your stomach and you manage to feed your baby with the help of your elbow. All you need to do is hold your baby sideways and use the head of your baby as if you were holding a football and bring it towards your breast. You must always keep a pillow on the side so that you have enough support for your baby and you do not lose balance while holding your baby. This position also works well for premature babies who are very small.

Lying On The Side

Lying on the side is an easy way to feed your baby when you are tired or when your baby is on the bed. It's an easy way to feed even if you're have undergone C-section or you are not comfortable with holding your baby in your arms and nursing. This is also the safest way to feed your baby for the initial few months. All you need to do is lie to your side and use your elbow to support the baby's head. Using your other hand, guide your baby's head towards the nipple and begin feeding. This keeps you comfortable and relaxed and when some babies need to drink for a longer duration, you will manage to do this a lot more comfortably.

Feeding Twins

Ideally, you should always feed one baby at a time even if you've got twins. But sometimes you can't leave another child crying while you tend to one and if both your babies are hungry at the same time, then the only alternative you have is to use the football hold for both. Use a chair that has an armrest. In such situations, you have to hold both babies on either side and feed them together. This takes a lot of practice so make sure that you have somebody by your side while doing this. They will help you with getting comfortable and also taking one baby at a time from you post-feed so you are able to get up. When you feed twins together, you need to stay as calm and composed as you can because you have to handle two children and that is not an easy task.

Breastfeeding Positions To Avoid

When you breastfeed your child, you need to make sure that you are feeding your child with precision and comfort. When you bend over your child to breastfeed, you will only block the nasal passage of your baby and it will be difficult for your baby to breathe while suckling.

Some parents choose to keep the baby's body and head in different directions while feeding. This is not good because it could damage your baby's neck and also cause them to choke more easily. When you nurse your baby, make sure that you bring your baby very close to your breast so that they are comfortable and are able to drink as much milk as possible.

Breastfeeding In Public

Just because you are breastfeeding your baby doesn't mean you have to stay confined to the house. Women are independent and have every right to step out even when they are breastfeeding and they can breastfeed the baby when in public. There is nothing to be ashamed about because breastfeeding is normal and is natural; and when you breastfeed your baby, you are providing your baby with nourishment in the most healthy way.

Know Your Rights

Breastfeeding in public is legal and there is nothing wrong with it because it is a biological need for your baby and it's the right food. Most women choose to breastfeed exclusively for 6 months which means they cannot give the baby anything apart from breast milk. While some women are comfortable pumping milk with a breast pump, there are others who choose not to use a pump and nurse a baby naturally whenever necessary. All you need to know is you need to be comfortable doing it and confident irrespective of what the situation is.

Practice

Before you head out with your baby with a mindset that you will breastfeed in public, it is always recommended you practice a little at home in front of a mirror just so that you get a fair idea of what a person sees when he or she is in front of you. Most women usually worry about exposing too much skin while nursing which is why they feel pressure to get confined to the home or go to a corner and try to breastfeed. You need to understand that when you are nursing your baby, your baby will cover up most of your breast so there is nothing that will be visible. You can also use blankets or a shawl to try and cover up while nursing your baby but this is something you will have to practice at home because some children cannot stand a fabric touching their face and will start crying, while others, on the other hand, are not bothered as long as they are being fed.

Choose Clothes You Are Comfortable In

It is important for you to stay as comfortable as possible when you are nursing so that you are able to do it more effectively. Front opening clothes are always advisable because you don't have to worry about pulling your top over your breast to feed your child. You should also consider investing in loose T-shirts because these are easy and accommodating. You can also consider wearing a tank top along with a cardigan. If the tank top has a stretching neck, you will manage to pull out one breast and feed your baby whenever required.

These days, there are a number of wraps available in the market that you can simply wrap yourself around with while nursing and this keeps you comfortable through the process. However, you can only invest in these things like a wrap if your baby is comfortable with a piece of fabric over the face while nursing. The reason you should consider getting a wrap is that you will never need to worry about the embarrassment of nursing and you can walk around while nursing if you have to.

An Easy Access Bra

While some mothers choose to wear a tank top without a bra, there are others who may not be able to have the luxury to do so because of the size of their breasts. If you cannot leave home without a bra, try investing in a sports bra that grants you easy access to pull up and down whenever required without struggling to reach for the strap. If you don't like a sports bra, you can also consider getting nursing bras which are easier to use. Nursing bras are easy because they come with nursing pads that provide your breast with a lot of comfort once you have completed feeding your child. When you invest in nursing bras, try to get a lower cup because this just makes it more convenient for you. Even with your bra, make sure that you practice opening it up and closing it before you go out in public.

Pick Your Spot

When breastfeeding in public, the one thing you need to make sure of is you choose the right spot for breastfeeding. No matter where you are, make sure that you are comfortable and you have your back well-rested so you do not hang over your baby. If you want to breastfeed in public effectively, always choose your spot beforehand so that when the time comes, you know that it is available to you. If your baby is fine with a wrap then you don't have to worry about getting prepared to breastfeed when your baby is hungry. You can always turn towards the wall and feed the baby so you feel more confident while breastfeeding.

Turn Away To Latch

Babies take a while to latch and this is the most venerable time for a mother because there is a lot of skin exposed during the latching on. If you want to feel comfortable before the latching on then use a blanket to cover up your front completely or turn towards a corner or a wall where you give your baby enough time to latch. Repeat the same when you are feeding and your baby has to latch on.

Smile

When you breastfeed, you will attract a lot of attention, irrespective of what kind of attention it is. While some people will be appreciative of what you are doing, others may look at you in a shocked manner while some may look down upon you. No matter what kind of reaction you get from others, always smile back at them because it shows that you're confident of what you are doing because you are concerned for the wellbeing of your baby.

Breastfeeding & Independence

Babies usually manage to switch between the breast and a pacifier or a bottle the very same day you introduce them to it. If you try introducing your baby to a pacifier or a bottle at a young age, there may be confusion. But when you try doing this post 6 months, you will manage to switch between the two conveniently and you will be able to transition from breastfeeding to other methods of feeding your child. This comes handy if you have to resume work and you cannot be available all the time to breastfeed. Mothers often worry about whether or not their child will be able to use a bottle or a pacifier and whether it provides them with the kind of security that they feel when they suckle on their mother's breast.

If you are planning to stop breastfeeding your baby because you have to resume work, you may want to introduce your baby to a pacifier and a bottle at least a few weeks in advance so you are confident your child is comfortable using this method of feeding. Babies will take a little while to adjust to a nipple that is artificial in comparison to the breast because your body is a natural way of feeding your child and it is designed in a manner to make it convenient for your baby to drink milk. When your baby sucks a bottle for the first time, the milk comes out with no control. This is because of the change in pressure. If you notice that your baby cannot drink the milk too fast from the bottle and a lot of the milk trickles down his or her face, then try to keep the bottle tilted a little so that the milk does not push towards the opening of the nipple very fast.

While some infants enjoy switching from a bottle to the breast, there are others who do not like the idea so much and would much rather stick only to the bottle or the breast. If you notice that your child is more inclined towards any one of them, try to make sure that they get comfortable with just that one method. If your baby finds breastfeeding more convenient, then you may want to stop breastfeeding for a while so they get used to drinking milk out of a bottle and do not crave the breast so much. To stop breastfeeding completely and get your child dependent on bottled milk, you have to wait for at least 6 months. Natural breastfeeding to the age of 6 months is highly recommended because this is what your baby needs and it works well for the development of your child.

Some children simply like to suck the breast for comfort even if they are not hungry and if your baby has the habit of doing this, then you may want to consider investing in a pacifier. Pacifiers can help them get some sort of security especially while they sleep because it feels like they are suckling the nipple. This also works really well when you have to move back to work and you want your child to feel comforted even when you are not around.

If for some reason, you cannot nurse your baby and you have to give your baby the bottle in the first few weeks of infancy, then you need to consider getting an infant bottle. If your baby cannot use the bottle then you may want to try using a dropper or a syringe to slowly feed the milk to your child. There are different kinds of nipples and bottles available in the market so make sure that you choose one you think your baby will be comfortable using. Invest in different kinds of bottles and a pacifier to figure out which one your baby likes the best.

Getting Your Baby Used To Formula

A child who is used to breastfeeding will take a while to get used to the formula for one basic reason - formula doesn't taste as good as breast milk and they long the taste of breast milk. If your baby is not really getting used to formula, then you may want to try another source of baby food that your baby might get used to. Apple juice with water is a great source of nutrition even when your baby is a few months old. Take a small amount of apple juice and mix it with water and try feeding your baby this juice at regular intervals. Once you start introducing other such foods, you can slowly introduce formula and other milk products that can help your baby get proper nutrition.

Returning To Work

Returning to work post-delivery is one of the toughest things for women to do not only because she is emotional about leaving her baby alone but also because she is worried about the wellbeing of her child. Unlike the olden days where women had the luxury of sitting back and watching their children grow, these days women are more career-oriented and need to focus on a career along with raising a family. There's nothing wrong with going back to work post-delivery as long as you prepare yourself and your baby for what lies ahead. Having said that, once you choose that you want to get back to work, you have to start preparing yourself mentally to be able to leave your baby alone. You also need to prepare your baby and learn to teach your baby some sort of independence so your baby can stay happy even when you are not around.

Set A Date

You need to set a date you believe you want to resume work because this will help you plan more systematically. Ideally, a mother should be with her baby for at least 6 months after delivery so that she gives her baby exclusive time as well as nourishment in the form of breast milk for the first 6 months. If you have to resume work before 6 months and you still want to continue breastfeeding, then using a breast pump is your best bet. However, if you plan on doing it post 6 months then you need to give your baby enough time to cope with external foods.

Once you have decided when you want to get back to work, you need to start preparing yourself mentally and physically and prepare your baby to get used to being away from you for long periods. Setting a date gives you time to prepare and plan exactly what needs to be done before you start working.

Check Your Baby's Weight And Monitor Progress

A few months down the line, you will manage to figure out exactly how much weight your baby gains each week and what is the progress that is required for your baby to remain healthy. If your baby is dependent on breast milk alone, consider using a breast pump to pump milk out and freeze it to be used later during the day when you are not around. If you do not want to give your baby breast milk exclusively, then you can also consider using formula. Try using formula a few weeks before you resume work so you can check the progress of your baby's weight and see how well your baby is reacting to it.

Get Your Baby Used To A Pacifier And A Bottle

If you are at work, the only way your baby can eat, it is with the help of a bottle. It's important you get your baby used to a bottle and also make sure that you know exactly what kind of food your baby prefers. Make sure to stock up on ample bottles and keep the meals prepared well in advance. Learn the best storage options for breast milk as well as formula. If there is someone around to prepare the formula then always try to get it prepared fresh rather than keeping it prepared in advance. Make sure all the bottles are sterilized and cleaned effectively. This is why more bottles come in handy because on days when you have to rush, you have a spare that was already cleaned.

Practice Staying Away

While you may mentally prepare yourself walking out the door and heading to work with a smile on your face, once you say goodbye to your baby, it's a lot easier said than done. Leaving your baby and going to work is the most emotionally draining experience that a woman will face and you need to practice doing that, so you are confident on the actual day. Try calling your friends and ask them if they want to head out to the movies and ask somebody to supervise your baby while you go out. Take a trip to your office if needed and check out your workspace. Ask your boss if you could spend a few hours working before you resume completely. This will give you a clear idea of how well-focused you are at work and how you are dealing with the emotions of being away from your child.

Supervision

Leaving your baby and going away is one thing to deal with but having somebody else look after your child is also a scary thought. Discuss with your partner the various options that you have with regards to caring for the child when you are not around. If you have parents or family members who are ready to look after your child when you head out to work then it's the best thing to do because you know these people will not harm your child and you will feel safe for leaving your baby with them. In case there is nobody you're related to who can take care of the child, you will have to consider two options - dropping your baby at daycare or hiring a full-time nanny.

There are pros and cons to both these options and it truly depends on what you think will work well for your child and his/her age. If your child is less than a year old, then they need personal attention and a full-time nanny who will be able to provide that. However, if your kid is a little older than that, then socializing is important so daycare might be a better alternative.

Secure Your Baby

If you're hiring a full-time nanny, make sure you have the house proofed with a nanny cam so that you can keep an eye on your child even when you are at work. While this seems a little extreme, it is always better to watch what's going on than to imagine things in your head. If you have family members in the vicinity, always ask them to drop in and check on your baby every once in a while.

Get Your Child Used To It

Whether you plan on leaving your baby at home with a full-time nanny or whether you plan on dropping your child at a daycare, you have to make sure your child is comfortable with the idea as well. Children blend in really fast but it takes them an initial 1 to 2 days to get comfortable with the idea. The best thing to do if you are keeping a nanny is to invite the nanny to come to stay over in your presence. You can explain exactly what needs to be done during the course of the day and get the nanny used to your child's routine. Let your child get familiar with them and let the nanny and your child spend some quality time alone. This will help your nanny gain confidence in taking care of your child. If you plan on leaving your baby at daycare, start with a shorter time span and gradually increase them to the hours you will be leaving your child there.

Figure Out If You Are Truly Ready

Once you have done all of this, always sit back and question yourself with regard to your decision and whether you are comfortable moving ahead with your plan. Make a list of everything you want to do to keep your baby happy and get it all ticked off before you get back to work. If you believe that your child needs a little more time with you, do not hesitate to get an extension. There is no denying that a mother knows what's best for her child so if you feel you need more time, always give your child that extra time so that you help your child develop better.

Breast Pumps

If you haven't already tried using a breast pump, you may want to consider using it to pump milk out of your breast because this is one of the most convenient ways of making sure your baby gets fed even when you are not around. Whether you are planning on getting back to work or simply living a more independent life with your partner that is helping you raise your baby, pumping milk out of your breast and storing it is something you should consider doing.

Pumping Your Breast Milk

You do not need to wait for a long time before you start pumping. Some women begin breast pumping as early as a few hours into delivery because this ensures that your baby gets a healthy feed even with latching on issues and it also increases the production of milk in your body without letting any milk go to waste. If you pump milk regularly, you will never suffer from any kind of swelling or soreness in your breast because of too much milk accumulation.

There are various kinds of breast pumps available in the market so make sure you choose one that works well for you. Before you begin pumping your breast, clean your hands well and make sure that you use a sanitizer that has at least 60% alcohol so that it sterilizes the environment. Always use sterilized bottles and sterilize the pump too before you use it. If your breast has a lot of milk, it will automatically start pumping out. If you need a little assistant, always try to think about your baby and apply warm and moist clothes to your breast to ease the flow. A gentle massage can also assist. When pumping out breast milk, relax as much as possible and get as much milk out of your breast as you can so that you can store it for your baby.

Storage Of Breast Milk

It is very important to understand how to store breast milk, otherwise, all your pumping efforts will go to waste. You can keep breast milk at room temperature for up to 24 hours once you have pumped it, but if your baby is not going to consume the milk within that time, the best thing to do would be to keep it in a refrigerator. Refrigerated breast milk can stay fresh for up to 4 days of pumping. You can also choose to freeze it and take it out whenever you need it. You get breast milk storing bags that are made specifically to freeze human milk. Make sure to purchase plenty of these bags and seal them properly before keeping them in the fridge. Always make sure to mark dates on the breast milk that you have kept in the freezer so you do not use any milk that is stored for over 4 days.

Freezing Breast Milk

Understand the procedure for freezing breast milk so you do not let any of the milk go to waste. When purchasing breast milk in storage bags, always try to look for smaller bags so that your baby is able to consume one pouch while feeding instead of having two thirds and then feeling full. When filling a bag with breast milk, always leave a little space at the top of the bag because each item tends to expand when it freezes and the last thing you want is for the bag to explode when frozen. Always seal the back carefully to ensure that no external elements enter the milk while in the freezer.

Thawing Breast Milk

Before you feed your baby breast milk that has been extracted by a pump, you need to bring it back to room temperature. When choosing a bag of milk that you want to get out of the freezer, always look for the one that is marked the oldest. If you tend to use a breast pump multiple times a day, always enter the time as well as the date when it was extracted so you get the oldest bag fast.

While you do not have to warm up the breast milk, you need to make sure it's not too cold because this could cause your baby to catch a cold. You can leave this milk outside for a few hours so that you can use it directly without having to worry about warming it up. Once you have taken out a bag of milk from the freezer, it is best not to freeze the milk again. Try to use it within 24 hours of being outside the freezer. If it is inside the fridge, leave it outside for 2 hours at room temperature.

The more you pump milk out of your breast, the better the production of milk and it also helps the baby to learn to be independent. This works really well if you have to leave your baby at daycare, with a nanny or even if you have to head out for a couple of hours without your baby.

Breast Versus Bottle

Most mothers who give birth choose to breastfeed the baby unless there is a medical reason or some important reason why they choose not to breastfeed. In my opinion, if you can breastfeed, it is something you should definitely do at least for the first 6 months because this is a great tool to assist in developing a sleep routine for a baby, and it helps your baby feel very secure which helps to incorporate independence. Although lots of parents believe that breastfeeding will lead to dependence, a child that is breastfed, in the opposite, turns out to be more secure and independent. You don't have to breastfeed your baby all the time. You can always use a breast pump so that your partner can assist you with feeding habits from time to time. The reason I recommend breast milk is because it is healthier than formula, and if you can nurse your baby, then there's no reason why you shouldn't. For all those mothers out there, I want you to know that not only does breastfeeding help your baby develop better, but it is also a great way to get into shape. If you've been contemplating whether or not to do it, I highly encourage you to do it.

Although a lot of mothers believe that it is extremely stressful to nurse a newborn because of their feeding habits, the truth is that it's not going to be that difficult once you come up with a plan. So all you need to do is think about your child's needs, and then you will be good to go. Breastfed babies actually tend to sleep a lot better in comparison to formula-fed babies because of the security and the comfort they get during the process of breastfeeding.

Feeding at Night

For the first 6 weeks, your doctor is going to recommend that you feed your baby many times a day; this means every other hour, even at night. While you may feel that overfeeding your baby is wrong, this food is healthy for your baby and important for their development.

Babies tend to start crying and mimicking the sucking action when they are hungry. As I said, the first few weeks are going to be erratic, and it is going to be difficult for you to understand your baby's routine because your baby is trying to adapt to their new environment all of a sudden. The reason it is important for you to nurse every two hours is because this helps to increase your milk supply; once you have a substantial amount of milk forming in your breast, not only will you be able to use a breast pump more conveniently, but you will also be able to come up with a feeding routine without worrying about whether or not you will be able to nurse your baby.

A lot of mothers believe that just because the baby is awake at night, it means that the baby is hungry; however, that's not always true. Sometimes children just want to play around at night, so make sure that you check what's up with your kid before trying to feed them.

6 Weeks to 4 Months
After the initial 6 weeks, things get a lot easier, and you will start to recognize a routine with your baby. This is when you should decide what kind of feeding habit you would like your baby to adopt. By the sixth week, the number of times to feed a baby at night will reduce, and your baby will be able to sleep more effectively and for longer durations. This is when your routine will start to fall into place, and your baby will begin to understand what's happening on a daily basis. It's around this time that you have to also understand that while you decrease the amount of food your baby consumes at night, you have to compensate for that amount of food during the day because the calories that your baby needs to consume should still remain the same.

During the second and the third month, you will not be feeding your baby multiple times at night, and sometimes you will only have to wake up about two times to get your baby back to sleep.

Besides feeding, you can also take up other methods of soothing to help your baby sleep; this might also be a great time to let your child learn how to self soothe. During the third to the fifth month, parents get really confused because they notice that their baby is up during the night more often. There is no need for you to worry if your baby is awake more often than you expect during the night because it is around this month when your child learns to play and gets excited at random things.

If you have chosen to give your baby the bottle instead of breast milk for any reason whatsoever, the fundamental feeding habits stay the same.

Cluster Feeding

A lot of parents tend to feed their baby more food several hours before the baby goes to bed so that the baby is able to digest their food better so that there are no problems while they are sleeping. If you are still breastfeeding your baby, then it might be a good idea to extract milk using a pump and give the baby the bottle a couple of times, choosing to breastfeed only when necessary. While you can still give your baby breast milk, constantly putting them to the breast will make them want only breast milk, and breaking the habit, later on, can get difficult. The reason you should pump milk at specific hours is that it then trains your body to produce less milk during the night, and this will increase your comfort level and help you sleep better.

Introducing the Bottle

If you have decided to reduce the number of breastmilk feeds that you give your baby, then you might also like to incorporate a formula; however, you might not want to do it all at once. Try to switch one meal to the formula, and gradually increase the number of formula meals you give your baby before they get used to formula completely. If you want to introduce formula, you may want to try after 6 months of breastfeeding because breastfeeding during the first 6 months is recommended; you shouldn't experiment with any other food sources for these first 6 months.

If you are having problems introducing the bottle to your baby, you are not alone. My daughter refused to take the bottle in, and every time I put the bottle into her mouth, she would start getting irritated and cry. Here are a few tips that I tried using with her, and I believe they will work for you too.

Slow Flow Nipple

Using a slow flow nipple to feed your baby is a preferred choice. When you are a parent, you are constantly tired. There is no denying that you would want to feed your baby as fast as possible so you can get a little extra time to relax; however, that's not a healthy habit. Some of the reasons why babies refuse the bottle is because it is very different than an actual nipple, and this is a difference they do not like. Breastfeeding allows the child to be in control of the amount of milk they want to take in, and that is what a slow flow nipple does. Most babies preferred this nipple to a faster one.

Holding the Baby in an Upright Position

When you hold your baby in a horizontal position, only the nipple has milk, and this enables your baby to drink milk slowly which makes them believe that they are being breastfed.

Encouraging

One of the best ways to get your baby to move to a bottle is to gently brush the nipple on their lips and wait for them to open their mouths. Once they do, put the nipple into their mouth so they can begin drinking.

Bottle-Feeding Timing

When you start bottle feeding your baby, you have to be prepared to feed your baby for about 15 to 20 minutes. If you are feeding your baby at a faster pace, it's important that you slow down because it may take a toll on your baby's digestive system and your baby can develop colic. Babies need to breathe in between swallows, so give them time and don't force them to finish the milk fast.

Babies Can Smell

One of the reasons why babies refuse the bottle is because it does not smell like their mother. The reason I highly recommend substituting only one bottle of formula in a breastmilk bottle is that it's easier to get your baby used to the formula in that way. Babies are a creature of habit and don't accept to change that easily. Introducing one bottle of formula in between two breast milk feeds will make it easier for the baby to transition from breast milk to formula in comparison to abruptly changing from breast milk to formula.

Milk Supply

Most mothers are worried about their milk supply and whether or not their body will be able to produce enough milk when they need it and stop producing milk at certain times when they don't need it. Just like the sleep routine, your body also has a routine, and once you decide to pump out milk at a specific hour and you do not take out milk for the rest of the night, your body gradually reduces the amount of milk it produces at night. Similarly, when you start decreasing the amount of milk that you extract, your body starts to adjust and will only produce the amount of milk that your body needs to produce. The reason it is always recommended to make a slow transition from the breast to the bottle is that it gives you and your baby enough time to adapt to the change, thereby making it a smooth transition rather than one that is difficult to deal with.

Tips for Babies Who Refuse the Bottle

Kids understand the difference between breastmilk and bottle milk even if the bottle contains breastmilk. Most kids don't like to switch from the breast to the bottle. In such cases, you simply have to make sure that you lure them into using the bottle without forcing them to do so. Distraction is a great method to feed your baby out of the bottle. You can also try to imitate the breastfeeding position but give your baby the bottle instead.

Not the Breast

A child understands the difference between the feel of their mother's breast and an alien object. If it is difficult for you to get your baby to drink out of a bottle, you may want to ask your partner to help you with this. Let your partner step up and introduce the bottle even if this means you having to leave the room. This will help your baby detach from your breast and ensure that he transitions smoothly to the bottle.

Change In Environment

If there is a breastfeeding chair in your house or a particular spot that your baby associates with breastmilk, do not give the baby the bottle in that spot. Try taking your baby outside if necessary or hold your baby in a different position altogether to try to get them used to the bottle. I would take my baby girl to the window and hold her in my arms while feeding her through the bottle so she was constantly looking outside and was distracted. This worked like a charm every time, and she didn't even realize when she got hooked on to the bottle.

Try Out a New Technique

Sometimes your baby might not want to transition to the bottle, and that's where a pacifier comes in handy. When your baby is tired and playing in the crib, you can just try and put a pacifier in their mouth for them to get a little comforted. Then, give them the bottle after they have the pacifier in their mouth; this method may work out really well. This is because babies tend to drink milk before falling asleep. While nursing worked well for you initially, getting them to suck the bottle and sleep might be a little tougher. Using the pacifier and then introducing the bottle usually works well.

Don't Give Up
A lot of women tend to give up trying the bottle because the child was not getting used to it at all. You need to know that children take a while to get used to the bottle, and it could even take as long as a month sometimes. So you have to be patient and persistent in order for your baby to get used to a bottle. It will happen eventually, but if you give up, it's not going to happen at all.

Earlier, I listed how you can introduce healthy feeding habits to your baby. Let's take a closer look at the various ways to feed a child.

Child Chosen Feeds
Child chosen feeds, or CCF as I would like to refer to it, is a situation where you feed your baby when your child demands the food. This would mean waiting until your baby starts to cry or show signs of hunger before you feed them. While this may seem the most effective way to feed your child, it's actually not that effective. The reason why you shouldn't depend on your baby to know when they need to be fed is that children have erratic feeding habits, and if you depend on them, you will never be able to come up with a routine. Children are also always developing, and their thoughts and desires change with them. What may seem to be a hunger cry today may not necessarily be a cry for hunger a week from now. This means that you will constantly be guessing whether or not your baby needs to be fed, and this is something that will

interfere with the routine and the sleep pattern as well as the general development pattern for your baby.

You are the primary caregiver, and it is up to you to decide when and how you should feed your baby rather than depending on your baby to show you signs of hunger. This doesn't mean that you completely eliminate this method. There could be times when your baby is a little hungry or you have given them a small meal which hasn't filled them up completely. If you notice that your baby is crying constantly, then feeding them is something that can help. CCF is something that is usually used for the first four months for an infant and then again once your kid starts talking and can tell you when she is hungry.

Time Chosen Feeds

As the name suggests, a time chosen feed is a feed that is given to a baby depending on what time of day it is. A lot of parents choose this method because they believe it is highly effective, and you will be able to time the feed of your child whenever necessary. While this seems like a great way to feed your baby, there is one problem. You begin to follow a timetable, and you will lead a rigid and very stressful life, making you depend on the clock for everything. While it is good to look at the clock every now and then, feeding your child based on time may not be as beneficial as you think it is because there are various external factors that could come in the way of this method of feeding, and it could create chaos in your life. If you want to lead a simple life without too much stress, then I do not recommend a time chosen feeding method because when you depend on the clock for everything you do, it will stress you out all the time. I tried this technique for a week and got so frustrated that I gave it up completely.

Parent Chosen Feeds

Here is a technique I really enjoy. PCF or parent chosen feeds is highly recommended for a number of reasons. It allows you to live a routine life without interfering with the various surprise elements that you may cross paths with on a regular basis. It will help you follow a routine that is not that rigid, and you can always make changes because it's flexible. If you noticed, I have always spoken about different feeding times, and the reason this is important is that although the feeding time is varied from time to time, it does not affect the routine in any way. Instead of deciding what time you feed your child, you need to plan how you will get to the feeding. Taking them to the park and then feeding them, irrespective of what time it is, works better for them rather than following a timetable. This is because children are curious and love looking around. The park has a number of things for them to get distracted by, and this can help you to feed them. You will be surprised to see how similar the time patterns are when you choose to feed them after following a routine, and this is a foolproof method because children are almost always hungry when you follow this plan. When they get used to a routine and their body starts to adapt to the various things that take place during the course of the day, it eventually helps them. This is also the easiest way to feed your child, and you don't have to wait for them to tell you or to check the clock to decide when to feed them.

Chapter 3 - Development Of Your Child

What Is Good For Your Baby

Solid Foods

Transitioning from breastfed to solids could be difficult for a baby if you try doing it all at once. However, if you gradually introduce your baby to solids a little at a time, not only will your baby manage to eat healthier, but he or she will also get all the nutrients that are required for a growing baby. While you should not consider starting a solid food diet for your baby for the first 6 months, once your baby crosses 6 months you can switch to foods other than breast milk.

If you are not able to nurse your baby, then the best thing for you to do would be to start off with formula. This will provide your baby with the necessary nutrients.

Once your baby reaches 6 months, you can start introducing solid foods into the diet. It is always healthier to introduce fresh food as opposed to packaged food because this is free of any chemicals and it provides your baby with ample nourishment. However, if you cannot provide your baby with fresh food because of a busy schedule, then you might want to check out some of the best brands you can purchase for your child. When choosing baby food brands, always look for the ones that are free of chemicals and pesticides as well as organic and natural.

When you have just started transitioning your baby from breast milk or formula milk to solid food, start off something that is semi-solid like a smoothie or a rice cereal that's in the form of a paste. Babies that are small don't have teeth as yet so the last thing you want is to give them something which is difficult for them to swallow and could cause them to choke. When you begin solid foods, make sure that you try small quantities first just so you know whether your baby can handle the food or whether your baby is allergic. Give your baby a lot of time to adjust to the food and once they have adjusted, never give your child something that he or she may not like. Fruits are a great way to begin solid food for your child but make sure that the fruits are always diluted properly and you don't give them too much of it because digestion could be difficult with certain fruits.

When your baby crosses 6 months, you can start giving your baby liquids in a feeder cup and you can also try giving food in larger quantities. Once you begin giving your baby solids, you will start to realize what your child enjoys eating and he/she does not. If you are matching vegetables and fruits together and there is a certain flavor that your baby doesn't like, try to cover it up with something your baby finds interesting or enjoys eating.

The larger the variety of food you introduce to your baby in the first two years, the more convenient it is for your baby to eat food without a fuss during the later stages of life. Rather than forcing your child to eat something they dislike, try to give them something they enjoy. This way, the encouragement is always there and they will clean up the plate without a fuss. Always try to include larger portions of vegetables and fruits in comparison to meat but also ensure that you include a fair amount of dairy in the diet of your choice.

Understanding What To Feed Your Baby

Switching from breast milk to solids is never an easy process and as a mother, you need to understand what works best for your baby. While some children enjoy eating fruits, there are others who absolutely hate it. If your child does not like something, you would be happier trying to feed them something else that provides them with the nutrients you want them to get without a fuss. There are also various ways you can camouflage fruits and vegetables to feed them to your babies without them realizing it. Milkshakes definitely work well with children and they manage to fill up on these effectively as well. It is also easier for children to start off with liquid-based solids before the transitioning stage so they are able to swallow more conveniently and you don't have to worry about them choking.

When you start off on solids, try to start feeding your baby small quantities of softer food so they understand how to chew the food properly before you try feeding them something that is hard.

You need to understand that children are used to swallowing when they are babies and it's going to take them a while to understand how to chew food before they swallow it. The softer the food, the lesser the chances of your child choking on it and the easier it is for them to learn how to chew food properly.

Don't Wait Too Long To Start Solids

Parents are always confused with regards to when they should start feeding their baby food other than breast milk. While some mothers choose to wait for up to 6 months, there are others that could go as long as 3 years without feeding the baby solid food. It is always preferred to start your baby off on solids after the first 6 months because this makes it convenient for the baby to understand the different kinds of food that they can eat and also how to react to the food. If you feel your baby is allergic to certain foods, then give them very small portions and see how they react to it.

Don't Give Your Baby Bland Food

The biggest mistake parents make is to believe they have to give the children food that has no flavor whatsoever because that's what helps the child digest. The truth is while you have to avoid spicy food, you may want to consider adding a little flavoring to the food to make it a little possible so that your child likes the taste. If you have to eat the same thing every day, it will annoy you and you would eventually dislike that meal, no matter how tasty it seems on the first day. It's the same with children. Try adding a bit of variety with their meals and experiment with different kinds of things you could give your baby. You need to understand that once you start feeding your baby solid food, you have to translation those habits into your child right up to the age of five. Try to experiment with as many foods as possible and give your child a variety of foods they like. The stronger the eating habits as a baby, the more convenient it is for you to convince your child to eat a home-cooked healthy meal as opposed to ordering from outside and giving them fast food to eat.

Balance Out The Nutrients

For the first three years of your child's life, you have to focus on the brain and body development because at this stage the baby grows the fastest and absorbs as much information as they can. You need to give your baby plenty of iron, Omega 3,

Vitamin D and Zinc in order for them to grow strong and intelligent. When choosing food items to give your baby, make sure that you ensure all of these are covered and keep changing the meals to ensure you cover every nutrient that is required during the day.

Don't Get Them Hooked On To Sweets

It's good to give your child a chocolate every now and then, but try not to make a habit out of it because children tend to crave sweets more often in comparison to others, and they would like to make it a main meal if they could. If you notice that your child craves a lot of sweets, try keeping the sweet things out of sight and try to include more fruits that are also sweet but healthy.

Know Went To Stop

Every baby is different and while some children have a large appetite, others may not necessarily eat so much. If you notice that your baby gets full fast and does not show any interest in eating anymore, do not force your child to eat. Instead, try to give them smaller meals more frequently so that their digestive system works well and they can manage to take in the food that they eat. If you try force-feeding your child, this food is going to waste because your child will throw up all the food which gets stored in the body as unnecessary fat. When you feed your child, you should avoid outside food that is unhealthy and only feed foods to your child that they can accept.

Tips To Help With Weaning Your Baby

The transition from the breast to the bottle or a feeding cup could take a while and if you want to make this transition as soon as possible, you need to give your child enough time and have a lot of patience. Children do not like a lot of change especially when it comes to their feeding habits. When you first introduce your baby to the bottle, try it with the best breast milk that has been pumped so they don't find a lot of change in the taste and learn how to adjust to it. If you try to feed your baby a different kind of food, it will be more difficult for your child to adjust in comparison to something that they are used to in a new environment. Once your child gets used to drinking breast milk out of a bottle, you might then want to slowly start introducing them to external foods a little at a time.

Slowly Reduce Breastfeeding

Once you introduce your baby to the bottle and you know for a fact that your child has become comfortable with the bottle, you can reduce the number of times you breastfeed your baby and replace it with the bottle.

Keep Your Baby Close
When you are trying to get your baby off the breast and onto a bottle or solid foods, always hold your baby close and comfort your baby while doing this.

Move Around
Moving around with your baby rather than sitting still can definitely work in your favor because kids tend to get distracted really fast and they like looking around. When they do that, slowly slip the bottle into their mouth and get them accustomed to it. The more you learn how to distract your child while feeding, the easier the feeding sessions will become.

Give Your Baby A Lot Of Attention
Breastfeeding doesn't just feed a child and keep them full, but it also gives them warmth and a feeling of security. When you take that away from them, you need to replace it by giving them more attention and always being close to them. While some children manage to get used to the bottle fast, there are others that take a long time so let your child get used to a new method of feeding on their own rather than forcing them to do it.

Cognitive Development
Cognitive development is one of the major reasons why some babies find it difficult to sleep even after

they turn 4 months old. Your baby is usually aware around the four-month mark, and this level of awareness will keep increasing as each day passes. This usually causes a lot of sleep regression because your child is curious about everything around him, causing him to stay awake for as long as possible. The best thing to do in such a scenario is to create an environment around your child where she is not exposed to anything new. When they see the same things on a daily basis, their level of inquisitiveness will not be that high, and they will eventually soothe themselves to sleep.

There are various factors that could cause sleep problems with your baby, and you need to figure out what these factors are and how you can fix them. You also need to make note of certain points mentioned below in order to ensure that you correct your child's sleeping problems without causing too much disruption in their daily life. It is easy to overreact and do everything possible to ensure that your baby develops a healthy sleep habit; however, too many changes may cause other complications with your baby's health. Here are a few things that you need to keep in mind when you are trying to solve your child's sleep problems:

- Make changes to your child's routine to benefit them and not to benefit you. Your sole purpose should be to change your routine so that your baby benefits from it. You cannot force your child to go off to sleep at 7:00 p.m. just because you want to go out and party each and every night. You need to start being a responsible parent and develop a routine for your child that will help them become healthy.

- Avoid using stimulations to get your child to fall asleep. I know a few parents that try playing music or play the television for the child just so they can get tired and fall asleep. These stimulations do not work long term, and you need to find natural ways of getting your child to sleep on their own. From my experience, I learned that it is best to keep your child in a quiet and dark room. When you try to give your child the pacifier or the bottle to get them to sleep, they will start becoming dependent on this method.

- Avoid changing your child's sleeping position once they have fallen asleep. Always try to avoid getting a child to sleep on the couch or in your room and then shifting them to their room. If your child wakes up in a different place than where they fell asleep, they will usually feel startled and cry out for help.

- If you are adopting a waiting approach for your child, then you need to make sure that you do not start when they are too young. The waiting approach refers to holding back your urge to run towards the baby the minute you hear him or her cry. A parent should hold back for two minutes before they decide whether or not their baby needs attention. If a baby really needs you, they will continue crying beyond two minutes. If not, they will go back to sleep. Most children learn to fall asleep on their own once they reach the four-month mark. Forcing your child to sleep through the night is not advisable because most newborn babies do not sleep through the night. The sleep of a newborn is broken into various small maps, and you need to find out the sleeping pattern in order to solve any problems with your child's sleep.

- If your child has learned to fall asleep on their own but cannot go back to sleep if they wake up in the middle of the night, then you need to start focusing on that aspect rather than getting them to fall asleep at the start of the night.

- If you are a two-parent household, then you need to make sure that both of you share the responsibilities. It is very easy for partners to divide tasks in the household based on convenience; however, that is the wrong technique. You need to share responsibilities with one another because swapping duties with each other can make the task easier, and you will not feel stressed if you do not have to put your child to sleep every single night.

- Avoid waiting too long before you respond to your child's cries because some children tend to throw up or fall sick if the parents do not arrive soon.

- Under most circumstances, avoid using a sitter to put your child to sleep because your child will then get accustomed to the sitter being around.

Becoming a parent is an amazing experience, but it doesn't always go as planned. There are various problems that you may come across, and it's important that you keep yourself prepared for all of these so that you will be a better parent to your child and help them develop healthy habits. If you're worried about certain circumstances under which you got a baby, then here are a few ways to deal with these situations.

Premature Births

Most women are not prepared for premature birth, but the truth is that 1 out of 10 pregnant women will have a baby preterm. A premature baby is a baby that is born before the 37th week, and this means that the baby is a little more fragile and delicate as compared to a baby that was born full term.

Thankfully, there are modern methods that can help a preterm baby become healthy in no time, and if you had a preterm baby, there is nothing to worry about. Just make sure you listen to your doctor and follow their instructions correctly.

The pregnancy of a woman is divided into three terms. The first trimester, or the first 12 weeks of pregnancy, is when the fertilized egg starts growing slowly in the body. The second trimester, which starts after the 26th week, is the time when the baby starts to actually look like a human. The third trimester is when the baby begins to store water and fat in the body so that they can come outside. This is when the baby's heart, lungs, and skin develop and they learn how to breathe. If a baby is born at this time, then the baby is healthy and completely developed; however, babies that arrive before this will have a few problems and are considered to be preterm or premature babies.

Birth Between the 24th to the 26th Week

A baby born between the 24th to the 26th week is considered severely premature and requires close monitoring in order to become healthy again. Babies are usually born with underdeveloped lungs and could have serious health conditions, which is why they will need to stay on a ventilator until they develop and become healthy. Babies born in this time are also prone to more infections, which is why they need to be kept in a sanitized location. Some premature babies are also known to have bleeding in certain parts of the brain, which is why it is important to look after them closely and ensure they are taken care of in the NICU. A lot of parents are sure that their baby will not be able to lead a healthy life when they are born this early, but the truth is that with the right medication, many premature babies manage to develop into healthy infants.

Birth Between 27th to 29th Week

Babies born between the 27th to the 29th week are also considered premature and require serious care because these babies could be mildly or severely underdeveloped. Most premature babies have lung problems because of underdeveloped lungs, and this also increases the risk of infection. Bleeding in the brain is also a common problem for babies this small. Babies born between the 27th to 29th week need to be kept in the NICU for a few weeks to ensure they develop well and get healthy. These babies manage to survive when given proper care and nourishment. While a baby this small tends to sleep most of the time, some mothers are encouraged to spend time with their little one and begin nursing. This helps the mother and baby connect, and it also helps the baby to feel comforted outside the womb.

Birth Between 30th to 34th Week

Babies who are born after the 30th month are considered to be a little healthy and could have stronger lungs as compared to a baby born before the 30th week. While they are still considered to be premature and have the risk of bleeding in the brain, this risk is reduced considerably. Babies who are born after week 30 have stronger lungs, and the chances of survival are also higher. Babies that are born around week 30 have a survival chance of almost 90%.

Babies Born From 36th to 37th Week

A baby born between the 36th to 37th weeks is almost a full-term baby and is completely formed apart from a little weight issue. These babies have strong lungs, and the only major problem is that they will need to be treated regularly. No matter how premature your baby is, the right kind of treatment will help your baby become healthy. While a lot of parents fear that a premature baby will have health conditions all their life, the truth is that once your baby develops properly, they overcome prematurity. This is a temporary condition, and all you need to do is encourage your baby to catch up and grow healthy. Viral diseases are a big threat to premature babies. You need to take one step at a time to give them the right medication so that there are no health complications.

While some premature babies may need to be put on a feeding tube initially, they can then move on to feed on the breast or a bottle.

Babies are kept in an incubator so that they are kept warm and develop in a healthy way. It also helps the skin to grow in case a baby was born really early. A premature baby is very small, and it's difficult for these babies to handle the temperature outside of the mother's womb, which is why you may want to consider a warmer room even after your baby is brought home. Baby's lungs do not start functioning until the third week, so if your baby was born a little early, it is going to take your baby a while to learn to breathe properly. A little persistence and effort will pay off in the long run. A premature baby can turn out to be just as healthy as a baby born full-term, so don't lose hope! Miracles can happen.

Just like a full-term baby, a preterm baby is also known to develop a sleep pattern, so do not refrain from introducing a routine into your baby's life just because your baby was born preterm.

Multiple Births

Everyone gets excited when they are about to have a baby, and it is safe to say that with most cases that excitement doubles when they are about to have multiple babies. While multiple babies bring you multiple joys, there is also a lot of responsibility that you have to take on your shoulders. While triplets and quadruplets are not common, these days a number of women are giving birth to twins, so this is a possibility you shouldn't rule out. If you are carrying more than one baby in your stomach, you have to increase your responsibilities, and this includes understanding their feeding and sleeping habits. When there is more than one baby in your belly, the chance of premature delivery is also a little high, so make sure that you take good care of yourself. Since this book is dedicated to the sleeping habits of babies, let's talk about sleeping with multiple babies.

If you thought that you could follow a routine and give them food and get them in bed at the same time, this might not always work out as well as you would want it to because it's not necessarily the same for two children. While they may be twins or even triplets, their habits are a little different from each other, so you have to double up your responsibilities and create separate logs for every baby. What works for one of your children might not necessarily work for the other. You have to understand the routine of each child separately and plan accordingly.

When you have more than one baby, it can become difficult to cater to their eating requirements, and you may end up getting sleep deprived if you try to do this on your own. The best way to tackle multiple children is to start using a breast pump so that your partner can assist you with feeding the babies and form a routine effectively without taking a toll on your health. Sometimes when one baby wakes up, they automatically wake up the other one, and even if that baby isn't hungry, your baby will be crying and howling for attention. This is a great time to introduce self-soothing as well so that each baby learns to independently self soothe themselves rather than depend on each other. While you can keep them in the same room, it is highly recommended that you have separate bassinet cribs for multiple babies. Eventually, your multiple babies will learn not to wake each other up.

Traveling with Your Baby

One of the biggest fears of parents is about how the child is going to adjust to travels and if they have to enter a new time zone. Let's get one thing straight: your child has no clue about the hectic planning required to travel. They just enjoy being in the moment and even tend to enjoy the flight because it's comfortable and cozy. You don't have to worry about making a complete sleep routine for your baby when you are on vacation, but you can always follow the same things you did as the bedtime routine to help your baby go back to sleep whenever required. When you are traveling, it is important for you to keep your baby comfortable, so here are a few things you should try to do.

Keep your baby in cool, comfortable clothing so that they can move around easily rather than trying to make your baby look cute, especially for a long flight. Ideally, get your kid a pair of pajamas and a cozy t-shirt.

You can also carry a dark bin bag that you can stick on the window in case you want to create a dark atmosphere for your baby to sleep. If you are living in somebody's house, you can always ask them for dark curtains, and if you booked a hotel room, make sure to see if there is enough darkness for your baby to get comfortable.

When you are in the plane, make sure to take a seat on the aisle so you can stand up and down with your baby in order to put her to sleep. You can also invest in a portable crib that you can carry along with you so that your baby feels comforted and is sleeping in a similar place.

Your baby may take a while to adjust to a new location, so don't get stressed out about your baby not resting. Give your baby a little time, and he will adjust and be able to sleep well.

If you're visiting a new country and the time-zone is different from where you live, there's nothing to worry about. Your kid is less likely to be as jet-lagged as you are, and this means that it will be easier for your baby to sleep just as well even in a different time-zone without any problems.

Getting Used to the Routine

Kids may seem unpredictable, but in most cases, children get used to a routine and manage to sleep effectively while their mothers, on the other hand, struggle to fall asleep because they are worried and believe their babies want to wake up. There are a number of women who have told me they sleep with an eye open to ensure that they are always around when their baby needs them.

When you become a mother, you want to be a hands-on mother that is with your child all the time, which is not a bad thing to want. Whether your baby has come into your family naturally, through surrogacy or through adoption, the early months of having a baby are always sleepless, and parents tend to stay awake to make sure that the child is as comfortable as possible and they aren't sleeping through the child's quiet cries. You begin walking on eggshells, and you believe that you have to wait near the crib just in case your baby needs you. This eventually takes a toll on your life, and it does not work out in your favor because you tend to fall ill more often. You need to understand that after a few months, your baby is going to sleep for long hours, and the reason this routine is so helpful is that it's a foolproof method of ensuring your child isn't going to wake up before a certain time. This helps you relax, and you will manage to sleep more effectively. If you aren't able to do this, then discuss your problems with somebody and find a solution.

Sometimes mothers just need a little relaxation, and they will manage to sleep a lot better. I listen to some soothing music and read a good book before I head to bed. You can also enjoy a nice warm bath or go in for a massage. Spending some quality time with your partner is also a great way to relieve stress and resume your routine life all over again. Becoming a parent is a wonderful thing; the journey is more than fulfilling, but you will be able to enjoy it more when you are healthy and sleep better. Stick to my advice, and your baby will sleep well. Don't stress yourself out by staying awake. Turn off that night lamp and lay your head to rest!

Helping to Mould Your Baby's Brain

When your child is young, you need to make sure that you provide your baby's brain with enough stimuli to learn on its own. Babies learn from patterns at a very early age. The reason a child needs to do a certain task over and over again is that their attention span and their recalling capability is shorter. A 2-month-old baby will remember something for a couple of days, but a 3-month-old baby will remember it for approximately a week. However, if you go on repeating the same action over and over again, babies will tend to learn them over a period of time. By the time the baby reaches the 6-month mark, their visual cortex will have developed, and they will start associating certain actions with certain outcomes. Your baby will be used to social behavior in and around the house, and she will protest if she sees that you are changing certain routines. I tried to change my baby's sleep pattern over a period of time. It took me about two months to get a pattern in place, but I made it a gradual change rather than changing overnight. If you have been getting your baby to sleep at 6:00 p.m. every evening and you suddenly expect them to sleep at 7 p.m., it's not going to happen immediately. You need to move the clock forward by 5 minutes every night until they are accustomed to sleeping at 7:00 p.m.

Changing patterns takes a lot of patience, and you need to be smart about it. You think that your child does not notice a lot of things, but that is not the case. Children notice patterns and learn habits very quickly; this is the reason they are accustomed to certain sounds and sights at certain times. My child wanted her favorite bottle by her side when it was time for bed. When it was her sleep time, she made sure that she found the bottle from any corner of the house and brought it along to her bedside. That's when I realized that my baby was learning and was adjusting toward her sleep time.

Babies associate habits with certain actions and visuals. For example, if my parents came over, my daughter knew that it was only playtime, and nothing else would interrupt her schedule. She also knew that when it got dark outside, it was no longer safe to go to the park, and she would not trust me to step out. These habits develop over a period of time, and you cannot force them onto your child. It's an automatic development of the brain, and these patterns and habits will come naturally to the child. One advantage of patterns with babies is they learn new patterns and forget the old ones very quickly. As I said, if you want your baby to learn something, you should try to get them accustomed to the new pattern by changing it gradually so that they forget what they were doing a week ago. If your baby has learned a bad habit, do not try to stop it overnight. Take advantage of the baby's inability to remember things from two or three days ago. This will help your child forget the bad habit and develop a new good one.

Try to associate good actions with sleep patterns for your baby. If you get your baby accustomed to sleeping near a noisy window or on your couch, there is a possibility that he will not be able to sleep in a very quiet environment or on a different surface. I always ensured that I put my baby down for a nap in her crib rather than on any other surface in the house. She very quickly developed the habit of falling asleep only when she was in a crib under a fan in her room. It helped me find a routine for her and developed the best sleep pattern for both of us.

The First Four Months

The first four months are very crucial for the baby and the parents. Most parents feel pressured into developing certain habits for the baby within these first four months. This is the reason they start force-feeding a baby at certain times during the day or forcing a baby to sleep at a time when they feel that they need to sleep. However, the first four months are crucial for you to learn what your baby wants to do and how he will naturally learn. You need to let the biological clock of the baby develop on its own. It takes a lot of time for a baby's nervous system to develop and for their body to fall into a routine.

In the first four months, the baby will be very scared and will try to adopt any routine that soothes him or her. You can use this to your advantage and start using soothing methods that will get the baby accustomed to certain sleep patterns. When you start soothing your baby at a time when she needs you the most, then the baby will start trusting you and will allow you to fine-tune their sleep pattern. Always try and meet your baby's needs within the first four months; however, make sure that you do not over-help. We have already spoken about unhelpful habits, and you need to stay clear of these habits in order to let your baby learn naturally. The baby's level of awareness will grow as they reach the four-month mark, and you need to be aware of this. Your child will start developing a regular routine, and most of their actions will be predictable by the time they reach this age. This is the reason I have broken down most of the chapters in this book into separate age groups. One speaks about the first four months, and the other is about babies that are five months and above.

Chapter 4 - Healthcare For Your Child

Pregnancy is tough and stressful, and your first pregnancy is usually going to be the most difficult because you don't really know what you should and shouldn't buy.

While it's essential for you to have a clear list of what's important, you should also understand unnecessary expenses and avoid them. I've discussed what needs to be avoided in the next chapter, and this one focuses on everything you need for your newborn baby. These are the kind of things you can add to your gift registry to cut down on your expenses and make sure you get the stuff you actually need.

Baby Diapers

You can never have enough diapers because babies need a lot of them and they go through at least five to seven changes a day and sometimes more, which means a pack of 50 diapers won't even last a week. There are some amazing baby infant diapers that you can invest in or add to your gift registry, so you are prepared when your baby poops. Make sure to select one that is designed for infant skin because an infant has very sensitive skin and using a diaper that is not designed for an infant could cause rash and infection.

Baby Wipes

Baby wipes are just as important as diapers because when you change your baby diapers you need something to clean up your baby and using cloth or cotton isn't recommended. If you are adding wipes to your gift registry, try registering for a bulk packet because these don't go bad for a long time and they will last you a couple of months. There are a number of baby wipes available so look for something that is soothing and designed for sensitive baby skin.

Diaper Rash Cream or Ointment

No matter how careful you are, your baby will end up with rashes on their bottom, and the best way to treat this rash or sore skin is to use a good quality baby rash cream or ointment. Always consult with your pediatrician to figure out which ointment or cream is good for your baby. You need to look for something that's not chemical based and has all organic natural materials, so it is safe on your baby's bottom.

Burp Cloth

It is highly recommended you invest in a ton of burp cloths because your baby is more likely to make a mess during the first three months and you should always be ready to clean up later on. This cloth usually comes in a bundle of either 3 or 6 so add about two or three bundles to your gift registry just to keep some extra handy.

Feeding Bottles and Storage Bags

A lot of women need to get back to work soon after they have had a baby and in such situations, you either need to pump milk out of the breast and store it in a bottle/bag or prepare formula for your baby. Irrespective of which route you take, you will need a lot of bottles and breast milk bags to store the milk. Try adding at least half a dozen bottles and bags to the list, so you have enough time to sterilize them before you use them.

Quick tip - Make sure you sterilize the bag and the bottle before you store milk in it because newborns are very sensitive, and the stomach cannot handle anything out of the ordinary.

Rubbing Alcohol and Cotton Swabs

Once you bring your baby back home from the hospital, you need to clean the umbilical cord. In order for you to do this, you have to use rubbing alcohol and cotton swabs. This is something not a lot of people will tell you about, and most mothers are not even prepared about what needs to be done in order for them to clean the umbilical cord regularly. Make sure to ask a midwife or the doctor to teach you the correct method of cleaning the cord, so you don't hurt your baby.

First Aid Kit

A first aid kit should be at the top of your priority list even before your baby is born. I didn't realize this until later when my husband panicked and ran out the door to the nearest pharmacy to get one.

Your first aid kit should have a nose sucker, thermometer and basic medications your doctor has recommended for your baby.

Nail Clippers

While we're on the subject of a first aid kit, I'd like to talk about the importance of nail clippers specifically designed for infants. Cutting the nails of a baby is so underrated, and parents usually believe they can use any nail clippers, but this is not the case. I didn't realize the importance of a nail clipper until I had scratch marks all over my breasts because it's my baby's long nails and my inability to cut them with an adult nail clipper. There are safe to use baby nail clippers available that you can safely cut your baby's nails with. I highly recommend getting one of these.

Baby Formula

If you plan on getting back to work in a few weeks post-delivery, you need to consider getting your baby used to the formula because you will not manage to pump out a lot of milk and store it in order to feed your baby throughout the day. While breastmilk is ideally recommended for the first six months, if you can't give your baby breastmilk you can always alternate between formula and breastmilk depending on how hectic your schedule is.

Pacifiers

Most babies need a pacifier to keep them calm and help them feel secure when they're not breastfeeding. If you plan on getting your baby a pacifier, look for soft pacifiers that won't hurt your babies' gums. Try investing in a couple of them so that you can keep sterilizing and cleaning them from time to time.

Breast Pump

I can't stress enough how effective this pump was when I got back to work. While it is a personal choice, you can always try getting on manual one that doesn't cost so much and see whether it works well for you or not. The benefit of using a breast pump is that your baby is not dependent on you and you have a little freedom and time where you could just go relax and rejuvenate yourself.

Baby Lotion

Baby lotion is essential to ensure that the baby does not suffer from dry skin or any kind of rashes after having a bath. It is essential to make sure that your baby is comfortable once he or she has had a bath and al lotion will help soothe the skin from outside and keep it moist from within.

Washcloths

You need to have a few washcloths in hand when you have a baby around. It is important to know that your baby will drool most of the time and there will be a lot of wiping that you will need to do around the mouth and the chest area. It is best not using a towel because a towel may cause irritation to the baby's skin and this is where a washcloth will come very handy.

Baby Shampoo

You need to take care of your baby's hair from the first month itself. Apart from investing and lotions you also need to make sure you invest in the best baby shampoo that will help treat your baby's hair with care. There are a number of no-tear baby shampoo brands you can consider. You won't need to purchase a very big bottle because you need to use a very tiny drop each time you bathe your baby.

Baby Bathtub

Many people use the adult bathtub to bathe their babies. It is important you purchase a baby bathtub, so your baby has his or her own space when they are having a bath. A baby bathtub is not slippery, and it is safe for babies to use. Adult bathtubs, on the other hand, can be slippery and if your baby has the habit of standing up while having a bath, this could cause accidents and unwanted injuries which could be avoided with the baby bathtub.

Crib Along with Mattress

Getting a crib for your baby is essential and you can also ensure that you get a crib that will match the decor of the baby room. While purchasing a crib, you also need to make sure you invest in a top-quality mattress that will keep your baby very comfortable. The reason you need to purchase a baby mattress is that you would not want a baby to sleep on anything that could irritate his or her skin.

Bed Linens

Newborns are extremely messy when it comes to pooping or even throwing up after eating. While it is not advisable to feed a baby in the crib, if you have to do that, you need to make sure you invest in a good set of bed linens. It is always good to invest in three or four sets of linens so that you can keep swapping them as and when the baby dirties one of them.

Blankets

Swaddling a newborn baby is essential, and this is why you need to purchase blankets that will help the baby feel extremely secure and warm. Newborn babies need to be wrapped tightly because they are used to being snug in the womb. This is where a swaddling blanket comes extremely handy. If your baby is not very comfortable with being swaddled, then you can leave one hand outside the blanket, and the baby will think that he or she is not wrapped.

Clothes for Your Baby

You will have to invest in various onesies and gowns that will make it easy for you to change the diaper for your baby. Most of the clothes for babies these days are available with the button at the bottom that will allow you to change the diaper very easily without having to take out the top. Clothes are available in various sizes but always make sure that you invest in something that would fit a 3-month-old because your baby would grow very fast, and there is no point in purchasing new clothes every month.

Socks

A newborn needs socks all the time. Although one may feel that they do not really need to cover their baby's feet in summer, it is important because your baby's skin is very sensitive, and you would not want to expose the skin to the elements. This is the reason you also need to purchase a hat that will come handy during the summer as well as the winter.

Car Seat
A car seat is the most important item that you need to purchase for your baby. You should always purchase a new car seat as opposed to purchasing a used car seat because the used car seat may not be able to withstand a crash. The installation of the car seat has to be done properly. Look for a car seat that has excellent safety ratings.

Stroller
It is important to have a stroller; however, you can always combine a stroller along with the car seat that you purchase. There are a number of brands that offer this combination; however, you need to check the safety aspect of the seat before you go ahead and get excited about the combo offer.

Diaper Bags
This is something that you will have to purchase irrespective of how old your baby is. When you move around with your baby outside the house, you will want to carry extra diapers along with creams as well as baby wipes. Always look for a diaper bag that has an insulated section that will help keep bottles cold or warm as per your food requirements.

Don't Fall for These Money Traps

Every parent looks to provide their baby with the best, and there's nothing wrong with this. However, you need to learn to draw a line between what's necessary for your baby and what is an unnecessary expense. There are going to be a lot of new parents who will come and advise you with regards to baby products that they believe are must-haves. Here are a few of these things I believe are a complete waste of money and should be avoided.

Baby Wipe Warmer

I never really understood the concept of a baby wipe warmer because you don't have to wipe your baby's bottom with a warm wipe since cold ones are always preferred. Warm wipes could cause a little irritation on your baby's skin, and unless you are storing your wipes in the freezer, you won't need this warmer. If it is really cold in the city you live in, just warm a little water and dip the wipe inside the water before using it on your baby. It's economical and makes a lot of sense.

Baby Seat

A baby seat is something you need to avoid, and while it has become a really popular item to have in a household, it is best avoided. It is dangerous forcing your baby to sit even before they are ready to walk, and this could cause a major accident.

When your baby becomes ready to sit just use a normal chair!

Talcum Powder

Baby talcum powder has been really popular, and people are so used to patting the baby's bottoms with this powder every time they have a bath. However, this is best avoided because there have been reports of baby talcum powder being linked to ovarian cancer.

Baby Food Blender

A baby blender works just as effectively as your blender, and it does nothing different. You can blend your baby's food in your regular blender and investing in a baby blender makes no sense.

Expensive Swings and Rockers

Most new parents get frustrated when their baby does not sleep because they need to be held all the time. One of the things that most parents do is invest in expenses swings or rockers that they feel will put the baby to sleep. What these parents don't realize is the child will eventually start sleeping on their own, and the rocker will just be a waste of money lying in the corner of the room. As parents, you should take turns to hold the baby because this phase is not going to last long, and babies outgrow it very quickly.

Emergency Bottle and Formula
When you are not breastfeeding, it is always advisable to purchase formula because it will help provide nourishment to the baby. However, if you are breastfeeding and you do not have to feed anything else to the baby there is no point in purchasing formula just for the heck of it. Having formula around could even be a barrier to you breastfeeding your baby and this is the reason you need to keep it away for as long as possible when you are breastfeeding your baby.

Baby Shoes
These are a complete no-no. Your baby is not going to walk until he or she is about 7 to 8 months old. There is no point in purchasing shoes for a 1 month or 2-month-old baby because it is never going to be used. There are parents who spend hundreds of dollars on expensive branded shoes just because they want their baby to look good. Making such investments is of no use until your baby starts walking.

Baby Walkers
Let me make one thing straight - a walker will not teach your baby to walk. Most babies are able to figure out walking on their own. We should all remember that our parents learned to walk even when walkers were not even invented. Some babies learn to walk later than other babies; however, this should not be a cause for concern.

Forcing your baby to walk with the assistance of a walker is definitely not recommended.

Hooded Towels

Babies need towels however, they do not need towels that come with a hood. Babies grow at a very fast pace in the first year and purchasing a towel with the tiny little hood will be of no use in a couple of weeks.

Pregnancy is a long and beautiful journey that has its ups and downs. While you can try to figure out a few hacks to help you through your journey, you also need to remind yourself that every individual is different and what works well for someone else may not work as effectively for you. Take time to figure out your rhythm, and you'll get better with each day.

The journey of parenting begins from conception, and it's a role you need to live up to, every day of your life. While you'll enjoy it for the most part, for the times you don't - just take a deep breath and start over! It's not about perfection, but about enjoying parenthood and making the most of it.

Uncovering the Facts About SIDS

One of the biggest fears for most parents is SIDS. SIDS is sudden infant death syndrome, and this is usually related to the sleep environment and the sleeping position of the child. It most commonly occurs in children that are less than 1 year old. Most medical investigations have not been able to explain this sudden death phenomenon. In most of the cases, the child suddenly stops breathing, and their heart stops beating. 90% of SIDS cases happen within the first 6 months, and there are a few things you can do to avoid this risk. The risk of SIDS is usually noticed in children that are premature or of low birth weight. Smoking by the mother during pregnancy and no prenatal care are also a couple of factors that affect SIDS.

One of the major risks for SIDS is when the child sleeps in a facedown position. There are some doctors that will ask you to make a child sleep in this position if they know that your child is not at risk for SIDS. However, if your doctor has not advised you to do so, then you need to always make your child sleep on his or her back. If you feel that lying on the back for prolonged hours can cause discomfort to your child, you can also try to move her to her side but never facedown. Some pediatricians and also a few parents hear that if they make their baby sleep on their back, they might choke if they vomit in their sleep, but this has never been the problem. SIDS is a bigger problem than choking during sleep, so you need to make sure that your child sleeps on his back.

Another problem that may occur by making a child sleep on their back is the back of the head may become flat. This is because the skull is still forming and can take any shape if exposed to pressure for prolonged hours. To avoid this, try turning your baby's head from side to side regularly. You can also try to turn the crib away from the light and towards the light at certain times; this will make your baby turn his or her head automatically away from the light. As compared to the flattening of the back of the head, SIDS is a lot more dangerous. Your baby's head will correct itself, but a baby affected by SIDS will not recover.

By the age of 6 months, the baby will be able to turn from his back to his stomach, but at this stage, the risk of SIDS would be lower. You should also ensure that your child does not sleep on a surface that is not specifically designed for infants, for example, a water bed, a soft sofa, quilt, pillow or sheepskin. When a baby sleeps on soft surfaces or is tucked under loose bedding, there is always the risk of suffocation. Suffocation also occurs when certain parents choose co-sleeping over independent sleeping. When you are co-sleeping with your child and one of the parents is overweight, there is a risk of entrapment and of overlying where the parent may roll over the infant. As absurd as this may sound, there have been cases of entrapment that have been reported in the past. You can never be too sure when it comes to your baby's sleeping position, and you need to do everything possible to ensure that there is no chance of suffocation or entrapment.

Another major cause of SIDS can be cigarette smoking in and around the house. You should also avoid overheating your child. You need to dress your child according to the temperature in the house as well as the temperature outside. Overlapping your child in bedding and clothes will cause overheating, and this can also result in suffocation.

Chapter 5 - Understanding Sleep Patterns

The first year of the baby will bring about a lot of challenges, and you need to know what to expect in each of the months.

The First Four Months

The first four months are extremely crucial, and you need to set a proper routine for your child's bedtime. There are a number of parents that encourage self-soothing, while others opt for parent help. During the first four months, your child may not sleep through the night, but they will eventually learn to sleep for long hours if you establish good sleep patterns and develop the best sleep environment in the house. If you want your child to sleep at 7:00 p.m., you cannot play loud music in the house or watch television at a very loud volume. You need to get your habits in place in order to establish good habits for your child. You also need to find the right balance between soothing and self-soothing. Too much of either one can backfire on you. A newborn child usually has a lot of fear; this is why you will see most parents swaying and rocking their child. While this can initially help your child, they have to learn self-soothing in order to fall asleep. Overdependence on soothing by parents will cause sleep hindrances as your child grows older.

5 Months to a Year

Once a baby crosses the five-month mark, you will see a transformation in your child's mood. Some babies tend to laugh all the time, while others continue babbling from the 5th month onwards. You will start seeing the excitement in the baby's eyes, and he will start becoming aware of what's around them. This is because the frontal cortex of the brain is starting to develop. This will help the baby self soothe, which is why you will see a lot of babies moving back and forth in order to calm themselves or even sucking on their hand or thumb. Some grab their feet and put them into their mouths, while others slowly hum to themselves. All this is behavior that is triggered by the brain, and it helps a baby to self soothe when the parents are not around. Bedtime will no longer be a struggle because the baby will have found a rhythm and a fixed schedule. You no longer have to tiptoe around the baby because your child will get into REM sleep almost immediately. Avoid the use of a pacifier as much as possible because there have been cases where babies do choke on the pacifier while they are in deep sleep. Your ability to balance between soothing and self-soothing in the first four months will pay off from the fifth month onwards.

Sleep Timeline

There are a few things that you need to expect throughout the baby's life cycle. When the baby is a newborn, their sleep cycle will be very irregular;

your baby will keep going to sleep and waking up depending on the sleep cycle that you are trying to maintain for her. An irregular sleep pattern can be difficult to handle; however, since a baby is so young, you can mold the sleep pattern based on what you think is best for the baby. When the baby turns about 8 weeks old, he will start sleeping more frequently but in an unpredictable pattern. The baby will have one long stretch of sleep at night which will last anywhere between 4 to 8 hours and several daytime naps that will have no specific length. Once a baby grows old and reaches the 3-month mark, the baby will start sleeping more at night and stay awake during the daytime. Although the sleep pattern will still be fairly irregular, the lengths will be more or less predictable depending on what you are trying to imbibe in the baby. When the baby crosses the 5 to 6-month mark, they will be able to sleep for longer stretches at night. The stretches could last anywhere between 10 to 12 hours, and this would be a very regular cycle from this point on.

Swaddling

Swaddling is an important part of parental care, and you need to do it correctly. Here are a few points to remember when you are swaddling your baby:

- When laying a baby down to swaddle, you should always lay them on their back.

- Use fabrics that are breathable, and make sure that you do not overdress the baby at any point in time.
- You need to keep the room temperature cool in order to keep the baby comfortable.
- After you have swaddled your baby, make sure that there are no loose blankets around the sleeping surface.
- You need to stop swaddling your baby once she starts rolling over. This can increase the risk of suffocation for the baby.
- If your baby has started kicking a lot, then make sure that you stop swaddling the baby immediately. You can start using pajamas or blanket sleepers in case the baby kicks a lot at night.
- Make sure that you leave sufficient room for the baby's legs to move around and bend because this will help the hips to develop. When the baby cannot move his or her legs around, the hip joints will become stiff and cause a lot of damage to the soft cartilages. Make sure you keep the upper body wrapped very snugly.
- When swaddling the baby's arms, make sure that the elbows are bent and you keep the arms in a folded position on the chest. This is the position they took in the womb, and this helps with developing the joints and keeping the baby calm as well. Your baby will try to suck his thumb, as this is their natural instinct. You need to give them the opportunity to do that even when they are swaddled.
- When your baby has outgrown the swaddling phase, you can choose to go cold turkey or you can

start gradually. You can try transitioning with one or two arms out of the swaddle for a few nights and eventually take away the swaddle altogether.

Sleeping Practices

Now that we've spoken about the various ways that you can swaddle your baby and regulate his sleep pattern, I also want to share with you some sleeping practices that I believe are safe for your baby.

- The initial few months are crucial for your baby, so make sure that you share your room, except your bed, with your baby. The initial risk of SIDS can be lowered considerably if the baby shares the same room as his parents.
- I cannot stress this enough: you need to make sure that you put your baby on their back while putting them to sleep.
- When laying a child down to sleep, always ensure that you put them on a firm surface. Avoid using a mattress that is old or has been used a lot. Some parents even try using car seats to make the baby sleep; however, that is not recommended at all.
- Avoid placing any loose bedding or any kind of soft objects around the bed. These objects can increase the risk of suffocation and could be really harmful. All you need is a blanket along with a pillow and a simple sheet.
- Avoid placing a hat on the baby while they are sleeping.

- You can use a pacifier while putting a baby to sleep; however, once the pacifier falls out, there is no need for you to reinsert it.
- Always ensure that the room is not too hot so that your baby stays as comfortable as possible.
- Do not keep the room too still, and have a small fan that will keep a little air moving around the room.
- Always avoid smoke exposure to the baby and keep alcohol and drugs away for as long as possible - forever if possible.
- Immunize the baby as per the recommendations of a doctor.

Stepping Up Towards Responsibility to Achieve Stability

Finding the right balance between assisted sleeping and independent sleeping is important for every parent. In order to build a healthy relationship, parents need to make sure they do not overprotect their child or provide too much help when not required. Babies need to deal with certain problems on their own, and while this may sound harsh, it will only make sure that your baby gets stronger and more independent as she continues to grow.

Let us take a classic example: almost every child is afraid of the dark, and when you stay in the room with your child because he is too afraid to close his eyes, you are unnecessarily being too helpful.

Children need to learn to cope with the darkness on their own, and this can only be done with the right approach. This chapter will show you how I balanced the approach towards my children and helped them grow and get over their fears.

Helicopter Parenting

Don't get me wrong - all children need a lot of love and parental touch. The sense of touch and warmth of a mother's womb helps a child build trust and keeps them comfortable while they learn new things around them. You will see this with primates as well as other animals; children tend to stay too close to their mother while they are exploring the world. This attachment theory helps researchers around the world understand the development of the child through the different stages they go through.

However, there are a number of parents that misunderstand this attachment and end up codling their child at every possible juncture. You will see a lot of parents encouraging their children to stick to them even when it is not required. In such a scenario, the children will not learn on their own and will not be ready for the challenges that the world will throw at them later on in life. Independence is important, and you need to encourage this independence from an early age. Parents tend to swoop in anytime there is a problem, and this is what is called helicopter parenting. Helicopter parenting is something that usually happens at night, and this is when the attachment gets taken very seriously. You will see a lot of parents exhausted because they follow this helicopter parenting method. I also suffered from this when I had my first child; however, I learned that finding the right balance will take care of my sleep problems and will help my child develop as well.

Parents who adopt the attachment approach of parenting will often hamper the child's ability to learn on their own, which will even hamper the child's independence. Most parents do not realize what the attachment approach will do. Let us take a classic example of a child playing with a shape sorter. Children love the shape sorter game, and it helps develop the brain to make logical decisions. While the child may learn to eventually sort the shapes and put them in the right slots, you cannot afford to get impatient with the child and help them place the shapes in the right slots. If you help your child place one shape in the slot, the child will automatically hand over the next shape to you and expect you to do it for him. This is the same thing that happens when it comes to sleep. If you help your child sleep for one particular night, there is a very good chance that they will look for you the next night as well. This is when they start to get dependent and cranky. Always remember one simple rule: if your child is able to do something on their own, then do not take away the chance for them to learn to do it. Struggling is a part of life, but when you try to take away the struggle from your child's life completely, they will never learn. You need to know when to give your baby space and when to respond to their cries for help. You need to find the right balance between over-helping and under-helping. This will help your child to learn and respond to you in the right manner.

When it comes to sleep, you need to make sure that you do not adopt any extreme methods in order to put your child to sleep. Some parents try to adopt the under-helping method where they put the child to sleep, shut the door and try not to respond to the child at all. This is one of the meanest methods that you can adopt in order to put your child to sleep. You should also stay away from over-helping, like getting into the crib with your child or rocking them to sleep. Finding the right balance between these two methods will help your child learn naturally and sleep better.

Helping Older Children

By the time your child has crossed the 6-month mark, there is a very good possibility that she has begun to sleep well. While you will still be responsive to older children, you need to make sure that you allow your child the space to feel secure and confident. You need to have clear expectations with a child and make sure that they understand their responsibilities with regard to sleep.

The First Steps Towards Parenting

Sleep is extremely important for the health and development of a person. You can compensate in terms of food and exercise, but you will realize just how important sleep is to your body. A baby's brain has already developed the need for good sleep from the time they were in the womb. While a number of people may think that it is difficult to develop a sleep pattern for a baby, let me tell you that it is not that difficult. Imagine the amount of time you will have to yourself if your baby is sleeping on time. Getting a full night's sleep is no longer a dream, and I will help you make it a reality. You need to have a plan in mind if you want your child to develop a stable sleep pattern. If your child develops a healthy sleep pattern, it will help them learn and remember things much better. This was probably one thing you didn't know, and even I wasn't aware of it when my first child was born. My daughter was having difficulty sleeping, and when I consulted the doctor, he informed me that her brain's prefrontal cortex would not develop properly if she continued missing sleep. You are probably wondering what the prefrontal cortex is. It's just a part of the brain that helps with our decision making. This certainly scared me because I did not want my daughter falling behind with her grades once she began school. Most studies have shown that kids that sleep less than 10 hours a day do not score as well in their cognitive tests.

Another plausible explanation for your child crying all the time is because he or she could be hungry. If you are lost as to why your child is hungry all the time, it is because of what happened in your womb. When your child was inside your womb, you offered him or her everything that was needed. Your child would consume all the food and then go off to sleep. These were the only two activities your child did inside your womb. Now that they are outside, they feel a weird sensation in their stomach called hunger. They do not understand what hunger is, and all they know is that if they cry, they can make the sensation go away. The only way a baby can communicate is by crying, and the initial few days will be spent crying in order to get attention and to try and subside the hunger in the stomach.

Baby's Sleep Dilemma

If you are facing a problem with the sleep patterns of your child, then your child could have a problem. This problem could arise because of a disorder - emotional or physical - or it could just be a normal reaction to the things happening around him. Sometimes you will be able to detect that your baby has a problem, while on other occasions you may not realize it. Some of the most common problems that parents face are for example difficulty to get their baby to fall asleep, their baby waking up in the middle of the night and not being able to go back to sleep without her parents being there, their baby waking up very late in the morning, their baby sleeping very late or very early in the evening or their baby being extra sleepy during the day. For some parents, it is easy to identify problems because their children suffer from sleepwalking, bedwetting or in some cases even sleep terrors.

However, some parents do not recognize their child's sleep disorder, and they often call them lazy for being sleepy during the day. Some parents notice that their children are snoring but do not realize that snoring can also be a sign of a breathing disorder; if this is not treated properly, it can start interfering with your baby's sleep. If you do not identify that a child has a sleeping problem, it will eventually start affecting their behavior and their learning abilities. Every child has a different number of hours they must sleep to feel well-rested, and you cannot determine that number for them. All you need to do is make sure that your child is active when he or she is awake and does not wake up at odd hours every single night.

Your Baby's Slumber Routines

A person usually alternates between REM sleep and non-REM sleep. The amount of REM sleep that one gets depends on their age and also various external factors. As your child grows older, their REM sleep time will keep increasing and their non-REM sleep time will keep decreasing. When a newborn child sleeps, he immediately enters the REM sleep stage. When she reaches her third month, she will enter the non-REM stage first and then move on to the REM stage. This is the pattern that will continue throughout your baby's life. This stage 4 level of sleep is what most adults slip into after the non-REM sleep stage. Stage 4 is a very deep level of sleep that most adults would have developed by adolescence. A child also reaches stage 4 of REM sleep on a daily basis for a couple of hours. When you wake your child, if he is in stage 4 of REM sleep, he may not recall being woken up the next morning. Let's look at an example: when your child falls asleep in the car and you carry him back to the house in your arms, change his clothes and get him to sleep without him even realizing, this is stage 4 of REM sleep. Sleep terrors and sleepwalking usually occur during this stage.

How Much Does One Need to Sleep?

As mentioned above, there is no specific number of hours your child needs to sleep on a daily basis. However, there are certain sleep needs that you need to take care of depending on the age of the child. Let's look at the age groups and the approximate number of hours that they need to sleep on a daily basis.

- Newborns: Newborns that fall between the age of 0 to 2 months usually need about 12 to 18 hours of sleep on a daily basis.

- Infants: Infants that fall between the age of 3 to 11 months require about 14 to 15 hours of sleep on a daily basis.
- Toddlers: Toddlers that fall between the age of 1 to 3 years require about 12 to 14 hours of sleep on a daily basis.
- Preschoolers: Preschoolers are children that fall between the age of 3 and 5 years, and they require about 11 to 13 hours of sleep daily.
- School-age: School-age is usually between 5 and 10 years, and children of this age need to sleep for about 10 to 11 hours daily.
- Preteens and teens: This is the age group between 10 and 17, and children in this age group need to sleep between 8 to 9.5 hours daily.
- Adults: Anyone above the age of 18 needs to sleep for a minimum of 7 to 9 hours on a daily basis.

You should know that these numbers do not necessarily indicate a fixed sleeping pattern. These are ideal scenarios that will help a person get proper rest and feel rejuvenated the next day.

Getting Your Baby into the Right Sleeping Habit

Figuring out how to get your baby to sleep is one of the biggest scientific experiments a parent can undergo. Although there haven't been any tests to see how to train a baby to sleep in the best possible manner, a parent can definitely try out certain techniques that can help the infants rest better and encourage their babies to form healthy patterns. The biological need of a child is very different than that of an adult, and that's why they cannot sleep for longer hours without waking up in need of something. You need to figure out a way to deal with the biological needs of your child.

As surprising as it may sound, parents usually influence the sleep patterns of a child from as early as the age of 5 months. You can't just begin trying to influence your child to sleep better once they have reached the five-month mark, which is why you have to start as soon as you bring them home.

Once you understand the basic factors that determine the sleep patterns of a baby, it will become easy for you to form a pattern for your child to follow, which will encourage your baby to sleep peacefully thus waking up happy and more active. A sleep-deprived baby is dull, but a well-rested baby develops better and is more active and happy.

Co-Sleeping

Many parents encourage co-sleeping which is allowing a baby to sleep in bed with the parents. This is a highly controversial topic because while some parents believe that they should always keep their babies close to them and coddle them while sleeping, there are others who are completely against this practice.

Children tend to adapt to the kind of lifestyle that you provide to them. This means that if you place the crib in the next room, they will fall asleep just as effectively as they would if they were lying beside you in bed. There is no psychological evidence to prove that co-sleeping is beneficial for your baby or that putting them to sleep alone develops insecurities. Some parents are just more confident allowing their babies to sleep independently, while others still have the fright of something going wrong which is why they want their baby in close proximity to them. As a parent, you should be free to try out what you believe works best for your baby which is why you should choose whether you want your baby to sleep in bed with you or in a crib to learn to sleep independently. I personally believe it's better to leave your baby in a crib because there is a risk of hurting your baby when she is in the same bed as you. It also creates an uncomfortable situation because parents tend to try and sleep with the least amount of movement so that they do not get too close to their babies. While co-sleeping may seem like a perfectly healthy alternative to leaving your baby to sleep independently, you need to remember that patterns are something that forms in your child when they are just a few months old, and independence is definitely something you will want your child to exhibit from a young age.

Let's not forget that privacy is important to everyone, and children have just as much right to privacy as an adult does. If you form a co-sleeping habit for your child when they are small, they will more than likely want to stay in bed with you even when they grow up, and this will create uncomfortable living situations for the entire family. When a child gets comfortable sleeping in bed with you, they will not want to move out of the bed even when they are a few years old. This will also become a problem if there is a new child in the house because your older child will not want to move out of the bed and will still want to sleep by your side.

When children form a sleep pattern, they tend to follow it more rigidly than parents do. If you need to stay up past your child's bedtime to get certain work done, it will be difficult for your child to sleep with the distraction around them. When they have their own independence, you can always tuck your baby in and make sure they follow the pattern regularly.

Most children who sleep independently tend to have a sound sleep 99% of the time from when the lights are turned off to the time they wake up in the morning. If anything, these children will be awake for a maximum of 10 minutes during the night just to get into a comfortable position to fall asleep again. This simply means that it doesn't really matter whether there is somebody with the child or not. They will manage to sleep effectively as long as you train them well.

Instead of worrying about co-sleeping and making sure that you are there with your baby in the night, it is more important for you to spend time with them when they are awake. They don't really care about you at night while they are asleep because they aren't conscious. What matters to them is who is there with them to nurture them and care for them when they are awake. For your child to be healthy and sleep properly, you have to create an environment that makes your child confident and feel secure to be able to sleep independently. Most monsters that children believe in only exist because of the stories that are created by their parents. This is something you should try to avoid doing when you are raising your child, and you should make them strong and independent individuals who are able to face the toughest scenarios. It is the responsibility of a parent to take away the anxious feelings of a child rather than build on them.

Unless you have space issues, co-sleeping isn't something you should consider doing because it takes away the independence of a child and destroys the sleep pattern. Even if you have to have your child sleep in the same room as you, it is always recommended they have their own sleeping space such as a crib or a bassinet so that they learn to sleep independently without having to have somebody by their side all the time.

If you are uncomfortable with the idea of your baby sleeping alone, then you should try to train your brain to understand that your baby is going to be fine sleeping in another room. Do not let your fear influence your decision.

If this is something you cannot do, then you should give yourself some time to try transitioning away from co-sleeping to give your child the independence they need. While this is going to be a lot more difficult for you, you should try to get rid of co-sleeping as soon as possible. If you cannot stop co-sleeping, they will not be able to stop co-sleeping either, which will be embarrassing for them. They will not be able to sleep alone and will never be able to go for sleepovers with their friends. Developmental issues begin with really small problems, and co-sleeping, in my opinion, is one of them.

Advantages of Co-Sleeping
- Always in close proximity to your child
- Immediate parental support
- Comfortable nursing solutions
- Spend more time with your baby

Disadvantages of Co-Sleeping
- Increased risk of SIDS
- Poor sleep for parents
- Parents tend to get separated (sleeping in separate rooms)
- Sleep cycles do not coincide
- Parents have to sleep at the same time that the children go to sleep
- Sleep problems start developing
- No privacy

There is no denying that the advantages of co-sleeping are very limited in comparison to the disadvantages. This is why you should learn how to train your baby to sleep independently right from the beginning.

Healthy Bedtime Routine

Performing a healthy bedtime routine is something that will benefit your child from a young age. Babies who learn to follow a routine manage to self soothe themselves and fall asleep much easier. This also helps them to get more sleep during the night, thereby keeping them healthy and more active. Children have certain wants and needs that need to be fulfilled at a particular time, and once you figure it out, you will be able to follow the routine much better.

Children are very quick to learn a routine, and once they start following those routines, they do not like change. The hardest thing for a parent is to stick to a routine, especially when they are used to living an erratic lifestyle that involves absolutely no fixed time to go to bed or wake up. Once you are a parent, the most important thing for you will be to stick to a routine because that's when you will be able to form a sleep pattern for your child that will help them self soothe and figure out when they actually need you.

A routine is something that you should incorporate on a regular basis so that your baby knows what will follow next and automatically tune their habits to do those things on a daily basis.

Your bedtime routine should be no longer than about 45 minutes to an hour, and everything mentioned on the list should be completed within that timespan so that your baby understands and anticipates what's going to happen next. If you try to extend this routine to a longer time, your kid will not be able to adjust to it so easily. When you put your baby in bed, make sure to say the same thing to your baby every night so they know that they have to go to sleep the minute you leave the room. This could be something like 'Goodnight,' 'Sleep tight' or 'I love you.' Remember to keep this consistent as it will become a part of your baby's routine.

Feeding Time Versus Sleep

One of the most important things to remember when planning a bedtime routine is that feeding shouldn't be the last part of your baby's bedtime routine. This could create uncomfortable sleeping habits. Babies may not be able to digest the food if they are put to bed immediately after feeding, and this means it could take them longer to fall asleep. Listening to soothing songs works well because it helps the baby to self soothe as they go to bed. Some children like to be swayed from side to side while others like to be placed on the shoulder before they fall asleep. Figuring out which way works well for your child is definitely going to be part of the routine. Babies tend to wake up when you go down to place them in their crib, but gently patting them on their chest will help them to go back to sleep just as effectively.

The Final Steps Before Bedtime

When you take the final steps into the bedroom, it could feel like you are literally putting down a time bomb, and your heart will always beat very quickly, hoping that your baby doesn't wake up again. If you follow the bedtime routine effectively, there is only a slim chance your baby will wake up crying once you put them down. The one thing you should remember while placing your baby down on the bed is to try and keep the light as dim as possible and ensure that the room is quiet and cozy.

Here are some interesting ways you can initiate self-soothing for your baby:

Put Your Baby in Bed When Awake

This may sound really scary, but when you put your baby down in their crib when they are awake, they will not find anything wrong with it. As opposed to yelling and crying to be carried, they will start reasoning with the fact that they need to sleep in their bed. This happens mainly because of the habit you've formed of placing your baby in bed to rest. Babies tend to pick up on routines, and when placed in bed when they are still awake and tired, they understand it's time to rest.

Increase the Time Frame Between Feeding and Sleeping

Try disassociating feeding just before your baby sleeps. Try getting your baby out of the routine eventually.

Learn to Ignore Certain Sounds

If your baby starts whining, grunting or babbling, you may want to stop yourself from going and scooping up your baby instantly because these sounds can be the start of self-soothing.

Use a Time Barrier

If your baby is awake and is crying, wait for a minute before you head to your baby because sometimes babies can go back to sleep after crying for about a minute. However, if they cry for longer, do not ignore those cries and head straight to your baby.

Independence

As much as you want to spend every waking minute of your time with your baby, you need to give your baby a little space so that you train them to be independent and you can go back to living your routine life. While in this stage, you want nothing more than to spend your entire life with your little one, but you should realize that it's not possible. It will be more difficult for you to separate from your baby when you spend so much time around them.

Tummy Time

When your baby tries to sleep on their stomach, it means she is trying to get comfortable with sleeping positions and is learning to self soothe more effectively.

Naps

It is difficult to understand the nap time of a baby initially, and this is why the first 4 months are quite confusing. Babies can sleep for as little as 5 minutes or as long as 3 hours. If your baby always sleeps at a particular time, then it's easy to understand that they will rest for 1 to 3 hours. That's the kind of time that you can give yourself to relax. Whether you want to take a nap, get a long warm shower, eat without having to hurry your meal or just admire your baby, do it. Babies tend to sleep a lot during the day, especially if they could not get enough rest at night. Even if your baby is asleep during the day, try to bring in a little sunlight during the day so that they subconsciously understand the difference between daytime sleeping and nighttime sleeping.

During the first four months, your baby is not going to be capable of sleeping for long hours, and this is the time self-soothing should definitely be introduced because it helps to encourage your baby to sleep better.

Catnaps

Short naps or catnaps are most common from the first to the fourth month, and this means the baby will be awake for a long time and sleep for short spans. This is usually because your baby will need to be fed multiple times or even changed. They tend to frighten themselves or startle themselves more often, and this causes them to wake up almost instantly. Once your baby has learned how to self soothe, it becomes easier for them to sleep a little longer. You will start to notice that they tend to sleep for 3 hours or so more comfortably.

What Causes Your Baby to Wake Up?

In case you were not aware already, you should know that all babies wake up multiple times through the night. Irrespective of whether the child is a light sleeper or a sound sleeper, there will be various stages when the child will wake up throughout the night. You will notice this in adults as well. There are certain stages throughout the night when an adult would wake up to roll to the other side or just adjust their blanket. These are the stages when you are not really awake, and you may not even recollect doing this the next morning. Your baby would also partially wake up multiple times through the night to do the very same things that you do - adjust their blanket, rollover or even grab their favorite soft toys (if you are comfortable placing them in their crib).

Some of these babies soothe themselves back to sleep, while others cry out for help from their parents. Most babies will forget what caused them to sleep in the first place, and they do not have the ability to self soothe themselves yet; this is the reason they look for assistance from their parents. If you have assisted your baby in sleeping by rocking her in your arms or by feeding her, then your baby will look for these actions when they partially wake up in the middle of the night. The same would happen to an adult as well. If an adult falls asleep in a comfortable environment and wakes up in a completely new environment in the middle of the night, they would find it very difficult to go back to sleep. This is the same thing that happens with your baby.

You need to start finding the right balance between sleep associations so that your child does not find it difficult to go back to sleep when they partially wake up in the middle of the night. Sleep associations are actions that can soothe your baby and put them back to sleep immediately. This could be the rocking motion of the parent, listening to their favorite nursery rhymes or even listening to a bedtime story. When you start getting them used to such sleep associations, they will want you to recreate the exact action when they wake up in the middle of the night. If you are not able to recreate them, they will never go back to sleep. Let us understand each of these associations and whether or not they will prove useful to your baby.

Useful Sleep Associations
- Soft blankets or stuffed animals
- Babies rocking their body back and forth on their own
- Sounds of nature or complete silence
- Sucking the thumb or the fingers
- Getting comfortable in their favorite sleep position
- Babbling to themselves in the crib while falling asleep

Sleep Associations that May Prove Unhelpful
- Rocking your baby or bouncing them to sleep
- Breastfeeding or bottle-feeding your baby to sleep
- Using a vibrating chair, a swing or any other similar devices
- Playing music to get them to sleep
- Using pacifiers that cannot be re-inserted by the baby
- Taking short car trips or stroller rides through the neighborhood

Sleep Wave
Sleep wave is a technique that can help you find the right balance between being too helpful and staying away from your child when needed. Let's

assume your baby girl is crying in her bedroom. There are various questions that will pop up in your head around this time. Is she fine? How long do I let her be alone? Should I go right now and calm her down? You need to remember that if you don't go in at all, your child will start wondering what happened to you and why you have suddenly disappeared. This will take away the trust factor, and your child will stop calling out to you for help. But if you go in too soon, your child will get dependent on you to soothe her back to sleep. This is where the sleep wave can help you. It will let you respond and also let your child know that you are not there to soothe her back to sleep. With the sleep wave technique, you need to pass the soothing baton to your child.

Babies usually find very sweet ways of falling asleep. Some babies lean their legs against the side of the cradle while others roll over to their belly. There are some babies that also nuzzle their blankets. Each baby has a unique ability that will help them go to sleep on their own. You need to find out what technique your baby adopts, and you will only be able to do that when you give your baby the space to employ the technique. In the sleep wave method, the parent needs to take on the role of a wave and rhythmically visit the baby's room. By rhythmically, I mean repetitively moving in and out. This can be a swift movement that will last about fifteen seconds. Your baby will notice this pattern every time he cries, and this will become a habit. When you move in and out of the room like a wave without immersing yourself in the soothing process, your baby will respond positively and start practicing self-soothing. This is one of the best ways for your child to go off to sleep, and the sleep wave method can be a great way to encourage self-soothing in your children.

Conclusion

Experiencing Parenthood is a beautiful emotion that can't be penned down in words. While the journey is exciting, there are a number of hurdles that new parents come across. It is important for parents to understand how to look after their baby in the most effective way and the right kind of food to help a baby develop and grow. Caring for your newborn and making sure you give your baby the best is vital. This detailed book not only helps you to learn how to nurture and nourish the needs of your child in the most effective manner, but it also helps you to understand the importance of caring and understanding your baby as well as what works for you and your baby. If you approach parenting the right way, you will be able to provide the best for your child and it will benefit you too. You will also learn how to transcend from being an experimental parent to a hands-on one with regard to all the needs of your baby.

Parenting is an ongoing process, and each day is a stepping stone toward learning something new. When I first became a mother, I had a ton of questions in my head. One of them was: 'Will I ever get to sleep?' There is no denying that the sleep habits of a baby are very different from those of an adult, and unless you get used to the sleeping patterns, you will end up getting frustrated and annoyed by your baby waking up every couple of hours.

Lack of sleep is something almost all new parents need to learn to cope with because your baby has different needs. While you need to be as sensitive as possible toward your baby's needs, you will end up with sleepless nights, and that could get annoying.

The reason I came up with this book is that I want all new parents to understand that it's normal for you to struggle to get your baby to sleep for a couple of hours before they wake up again. Sleeplessness is part of parenting, and if you cannot accept that, you'll constantly struggle to try different things to get your baby to sleep.

While it's easier said than done, there are definitely techniques that can help your baby sleep a little longer and also help them to understand the importance of balancing sleep time versus wake time more effectively.

If you want to get this done, you have to learn how to provide them with their necessities in a timely manner so you and your baby stay healthy and happy. I put together this book after a lot of experimenting and guidance from some of the best professionals I could find. I thought labor was the most difficult part of having a baby; the truth is the sleepless nights turned out to be way worse than I imagined!

Let me tell you one thing: once your maternal instincts kick in, you will not want to sleep unless you know your baby is resting. This means even if

you look like a zombie and you have erratic mood swings, you won't be able to rest.
It's important for a baby's caregivers to stay healthy and well-rested if you want to bring up the child in a healthy and positive way. I wrote this book because I've heard a number of parents complain about struggling and not being able to sleep, and I believe them because I was once one of them.

Reading this book will not only help you to figure out an effective way to help your baby, but it will help you to train your baby in a way that will help them when they grow up as well. I understand that there are a lot of parents out there living a modernized life, nothing like the traditional marriage. Whether you are single, in a relationship, married, straight or gay, this book is still applicable to you. From learning how to tackle your first breastfeeding experience to understanding what your baby needs and helping you with all the problems associated with newborn care, I hope this book has covered up all your needs and gives you everything you're looking for!

Do let us know how this book helped you by leaving a review. This will encourage eager parents to make the right purchase, also I get motivation whenever I hear someone who gets value from what I created.

Happy Parenting!

Toddler Discipline Tips:

The Complete Parenting Guide With Proven Strategies To Understand And Managing Toddler's Behavior, Dealing With Tantrums, And Reach An Effective Communication With Kids

Author

Lisa Marshall

Preface

If you are reading this, I assume you probably have been dealing with a lot of stress or anxieties that parents often go through, like dealing with the "Terrible Twos", poor child's behavior, tantrums, and all sources of common parenting problems. We love our kids so much, even though they sometimes drive us crazy. Their behaviors and actions make us worry that we aren't doing enough to raise them properly. I've heard a lot of mums and dads feeling frustrated that they are failing as parents, and I know, you want peace and quietness back in your home. You're not alone, in fact, you are in very good company. The good news is that you can get the changes you want. My experience proves you can actually turn things around to enjoy your kids and your time as a parent, much more than you are right now. I'd like to help you make those changes by showing you some of the most important tools you can learn to make this a success.

Here is the good news; most of the problems you're facing with your child's behavior are not your fault. Think about it, kids come without an instruction manual and, nobody trains us on how to actually deal with toddlers and preschoolers. They don't teach this stuff in school and when you're expecting your first child, you may have to take on those parenting classes to have an insight on what to expect; the session that teaches you how to hold baby, how to feed a baby and everything involved in taking care of a baby! Sure it's important stuff, but it's actually pretty easy compared to the "terrible twos". This is a big source for stressed parents, as you can learn and apply better ways to deal with your kids. There is only one real reason you don't have a peaceful home you want with your well-behaved children.

Number 1: Behavior is driven by emotion, not logic. This is the basis of the entire process. The behavior of any person of any age is determined by their emotional state. People act from their emotion and they later justify the action with logic. But little kids don't have the ability to use logic, so they act purely from emotion. Let's say that your child won't get to dress in the morning, or eat his dinner, or won't share a toy with a playmate. Your child mentally connects their behavior to some kind of emotional pain, and so no matter how many times you ask, they won't collaborate. Changing your child's emotional state is the key to getting the behavior you would want to see in them. So how do you change your child's emotional state? I discovered some very specific language patterns to make it easier for your child to feel good about the kind of behavior you would want them to display. Once they feel good about it, the behavioral changes follow instantly. I have seen so many parents trying to use logic on their children; "If you eat that cookie, you won't be hungry for dinner," or "If you don't wear this coat, you will be cold outside!" This logic simply doesn't work. You can validate this by thinking about your own experiences with your child.

Number 2: We tend to overuse the word "NO" when we talk to our kids. You remember the story of the boy who cried "wolf" many times, right? When a parent cries out "no" to every little thing, kids stop listening. People including kids are programmed to notice differences. If you driving down the road, you tend not to notice the normal behaviors of other cars or people walking on the sidewalk. But if a car suddenly comes to a stop or the child suddenly runs to the street, you do take notice because something is different. If you say "no" so often, it will be fade in the background, becoming ordinary as cars on the road or people on the sidewalk. The better alternative is to change your child's behavior without using "no" all the time. I will show you how exactly you can do this using language techniques that seem almost magical and almost too easy!

Number 3: If you want to have any chance at all influencing your child's behavior, first, you must have rapport! "Rapport" simply means having an emotional connection with another person. This is why when strangers are talking about the weather or gasoline prices, they are consciously making general comments they know the other person will agree with. The agreement creates rapport. It's a natural process that all we do in our relationships, but we also forget that we need to build rapport with our kids too. I'll show you lots of ways to create this crucial emotional bridge before you can change a child's behavior.

Number 4: Language is a powerful tool and there are a bunch of tactics you need to learn to create occurrences you want. Here a specific tip: Use positive language instead of negative language. Ask your child to sit down instead of not jumping on the couch. Tell him/her "Behold your cup into hands" instead of "Don't spill your milk." This is the opposite that most of us speak. It is scientifically proven that speaking in negative terms is insanely what you don't want. Who actually causes your child to do exactly what you trying to avoid? You want some subtle prove on what works for you right now? Okay, do not think of the colors of your child's hair right now. Don't think about it and certainly don't form a mental image of it right now. Seen? As soon as you are told not to do something, you at least think about it, so you can understand what it is that you aren't supposed to do. The difference is that young kids, unlike adults, don't have what I call critical faculty, which helps to process negative language. I've got some more information to share. Can you imagine what will happen if you install a powerful set of communication strategies within your mind? It's not as hard as you might think, and the effects are fast and powerful. How much peaceful will be your life once you know how to fix or even prevent most of these behavioral problems you've been dealing with. Would you love to start enjoying more and smile with your kids? One real thing you can understand is knowing that you're doing the best job you can to make their lives better. I want you to either experience the joy of loving and nurturing an emotionally healthy family life. It's entirely achievable because I've helped thousands of other parents learn how to deal with their kids more effectively. There are still far too many parents who share the same frustrations and need these solutions.

I think it is best to share my story with you so you can understand why I feel so passionate to share these parenting strategies with you. My name is Lisa Marshall and I'm graduated as an expert in communication psychology. One day, the university invited a guest speaker and that went on to change my life forever. The speaker showed us how to use our brain to make powerful shifts in our emotional states, he also discussed the basics of influence, persuasion and relationship building. This stuff really excited me. I would fall in love with this kind of argument, and I finished from school to become an expert in this field. After some years I met my husband and in two years, we had our first child. Since then, in that first moment, holding this tiny baby of mine, it always hit me that I had much more responsibility than ever before. By the time he was entering the terrible twos, I was pregnant again with my second daughter. Here, my training started to come in and things were bearing me so far. The challenges and problems we faced will end in a very typical way. This is where I found the idea that my knowledge in the relationships and influencing people could probably work on small children too. The tools just needed to be reworked, with the help of exhaustive research in the field of children, and for five years, I started connections and cooperations with many experts in this field. I took the time to take my communication skills and I adapted to them so well. I would reuse them for children, and what I developed is a unique effective toolbox for parents. I have always been a natural teacher, so after experimenting on my own kids, I started working with other parents. The results were truly spectacular!

Parents no longer felt like being out of control. Kids started to behave better as the results were fast, and best of all, the strategies I teach maintains a child's dignity and actually help the child to understand how to make better choices. I turned all of this in the book you are going to read called *"Toddler Discipline Tips."* The techniques you'll learn will work on any age group and not just toddlers. This book is unique because it is the only program that breaks up the science of communication and applies to the kids with the parent-approved emphasis on creating a positive influence on children.

"Children must be taught how to think, not what to think"

Margaret Mead-

Introduction

Congratulations on downloading *Toddler Discipline Tips,* and thank you for doing so.

There are plenty of books on this subject on the market, thanks again for choosing this one! Every effort was made to ensure it is full of as much useful information as possible. Please enjoy!

It's important that we introduce an understanding of positive discipline before approaching behavior as a whole. This book will teach you what positive discipline is, from when to apply it to how to do it properly.
Positive discipline is a new method that is used to look after babies and children in a different way by using a different point of view. While in the traditional discipline we speak of punishing wrong behavior, in the positive discipline, we keep in mind the type of adult we want to create and what would be the reaction of society to that mistake.

Thus, positive discipline is a form of non-punitive discipline that favors self-esteem, the independence of the child, and the bond between parents and children.

How To Act When The Baby Or Child Does Something Wrong

You must be thinking, if this discipline is not punitive, how will I act when my child does something wrong? Well, it would be just like when adults do something wrong. If you make mistakes in your work, you have to bear the consequences of your mistake, sometimes financial, sometimes moral, and whenever possible, you have to correct the mistake. So the child learns to correct something that he or she has done wrong.

So if your child hits another child, for example, applying positive discipline will teach the child to understand the problems that this has caused to the other child. The child has to learn to think of other people, to have empathy. Based on that empathy, you need to teach the child to see their mistakes and correct them whenever possible. It has no punishment, and it has no scolding, but everything depends on the patience of the parents.

Of course, this question of understanding the consequences of their mistakes applies to older children as well. In the case of babies, it is different. At that age, there is not much language. However, parents can start saying short sentences, like 'no, that hurts.' If the baby wants something that he or she cannot have, you need to take the object away from the line of sight so that it stops being the focus. If the baby cries because of this, parents should comfort the child but under no circumstances should they deliver the object to the child and let them have what was forbidden. When the baby is one year and a few months old, they already understand what the adults say. So parents can better explain why something cannot be done. Thus, positive discipline from this age is made up of many conversations and explanations about why certain things cannot be done.

When the child does something that the parents did not like, they should never say things like: you are a pest. Parents should make it clear that they did not like the child's attitude by saying something like: It is not cool to beat your friend because it hurts him. This method has very firm limits and at the same time, offers freedom to the child. It is similar to society, where there are general laws, but people are free.

How To Act When The Baby Or Child Does Something Right

In traditional discipline, when the child does something right, the parents usually show appreciation. However, when he or she does something wrong, the parents express displeasure. In positive discipline, it is different. It's important that parents try to show that they have noticed good behavior and praise it. It is also important to praise the effort of the child.

When To Begin With Positive Discipline

During the baby's early months, there is little point in applying positive discipline. From around 8 or 9 months, the baby has a developmental leap and learns to communicate by crying. It's a complicated phase because until this point there was no action of disciplining the child and now they insist on what they want. So from this point on, we can apply positive discipline.

Tips For Applying Positive Discipline

One of the most important tips for applying positive discipline is to never lie to the child. For example: if your child wants a cookie, but you do not want to give him or her that cookie, do not say that there is no cookie in order to avoid explanations. You also have to avoid bribery and blackmail because if you do that, the child always screams and cries. If the rule exists, it has to be valid.

Another great tip is to think well before saying no. After all, in this method, it is not acceptable that parents change their mind after the child's insistence. Parents have to take the blame for their own behavior. You must lead by example.

Benefits Of Positive Discipline

Positive discipline helps children to become creative adults. In this method, we do not punish the error, but rather correct it. As opposed to punishment, that creates in children the fear of making mistakes.

The child's self-esteem is stimulated with positive discipline. In this method, we encourage learning to reward achievements. For example, if your child wants a bike and you give it to him or her the same day, the child has nothing to wait for. So it's interesting that parents set a date for him or her to get the bike, for example, her birthday.

Positive discipline has a number of positive effects on the confidence of the child. This book will help you understand how to discipline your child without using fear as a weapon.

Chapter 1: Understanding Toddler Behavior

Toddlers are difficult to understand for even the most patient and nurturing adult. Keeping a positive outlook and going easy on yourself on the difficult days is imperative. What if your child bites his little friend, or throws food on the floor and starts yelling? How do we prepare ourselves to deal with this moment? The idea, of course, is to always opt for the path of a good education. To do this, we talked to some experts, who suggested ways to deal with children for bad behaviors.

Deciphering child behavior is not an easy task for parents. The quest for answers often runs counter to the way they raise their children, the amount of "no" they can say to them, within the limits they can impose. Often, adults sense how they should act, but the fear of frustrating children ultimately results in resignation. Indeed, children have standard attitudes in every stage of life, but that does not mean that adults have to follow orders and accept all attacks as something natural in the development process. To help parents act during difficult times, we sought out child education and behavioral experts who suggested ways to understand toddler behavior.

Up To 2 Years Old

1. My child has the habit of biting people. How do we teach him that this is wrong? It's expected by professionals who deal with children that they will bite until they are 3 or 4 years old, but adults cannot allow them to bite, because it hurts and it's wrong. By the time your child bites a classmate or anyone else, the professional counsels the good old eye-to-eye conversation. Stay at the same height as the child and speak firmly that this cannot and should not happen because it hurts. Parents have to make it clear that they do not approve of this behavior because even though they do not have clear notions of right and wrong, they cannot do everything they want. This does not mean that behavior does not repeat itself, but every time it occurs, it is necessary to make your position clear.

2. What do I do to stop my child from crying? Children below 2 years of age have no resourceful means of communicating, so constant crying indicates discomfort, physical or emotional, that needs to be investigated by the doctor. As the baby does not know how to speak, they use crying to demonstrate that they're suffering. From the age of 2, however, the child already realizes how he or she can manipulate their parents and uses crying to try to get what they want. I believe that one of the ways to help your child to learn to cope with frustration is by disregarding their desires when they come along with the temper tantrums.

3. How should I act in the face of a raging attack by my child in public places or if he kicks when he is not served?

The suggestion here is to try to prevent the child from seeing your frustration. If necessary, you should hug the child from behind to contain him or her. This way, you do not show your annoyance. Tell them that their behavior is wrong, that you do not approve of the way they act. If it does not work and he or she is not in danger, I suggest that the parents move away and allow the child to get their energy out. Most people have spent time with children and will have some understanding of what you are going through. Do not feel embarrassed or like a failure as a parent. We've all been there. Once your child realizes that their behavior will not get them the desired result, he or she will stop.

4. My son loves to slap his face and pull people's hair. What should I tell him at those times?

Though there are times when this can be amusing, it's best to never give that kind of attention to this type of thing. The behavior should not be tolerated. Hold the baby's hand(do not laugh or make a face that shows you become sad when this happens). It is by observing the reaction of others that children learn to interpret feelings and develop empathy for others. Always speak of your feelings. Never use negative terms about your child like bad or ugly. And do not fall into the trap of spanking. If you do, you will be reinforcing the learning of physical aggression, which is a bad example.

5. When displeased, my son begins to scream. How can I show that this is wrong?
Is this child learning this behavior from you? If you cannot control yourself, the child may just be repeating what he sees. Think about it. Accepting frustrations is a major difficulty nowadays for parents and children. How often do you get frustrated that you do not earn more or that you are not recognized at work as you should?

With an older child, you can pretend you do not know and leave her screaming on her own. If you leave, you will see that she will not repeat the same thing again. In the case of small ones, the solution is to try to calm them down. Hug the child from behind, be quiet, and make sounds like 'Ssshhhh' in her ear.

6. My 1-year-old son, when irritated, bangs his head on the floor or wall. How should I act?
If the child is at risk of injury, you must hold the child and stop the action by hugging from behind. It is worth trying the technique of making the 'Ssshhhh' sound in the ear and asking him to calm down. If none of this works and he continues to make this action, you must seek the help of a doctor. Self-harm is not acceptable behavior and can indicate serious mental disorders and needs an assessment from a psychiatrist.

7. My 1-year-old and 2-month-old baby test my patience every day. Should I show him what he

can or cannot do? Does he already understand the concept of right and wrong?

He may not distinguish between right and wrong, but at this age, he begins to perceive inconsistencies. How often do children at this stage test their parents? When they do something, they look at them and hear the no; they do it again until the father or mother asks to stop the act. And they repeat this many times, demonstrating that they have a certain notion of what is important.

Over 2 Years Old

1. My daughter is throwing tantrums in public places, such as shopping. How shall I rebuke her? Children with this kind of recurring behavior have no limits and may feel devoid of affection and attention. This is not to say that parents do not love them, just that they may not know how to demonstrate it. Another reason is that many parents fail to understand the role of frustration and fear. They may feel they're not deserving of love unless they do everything for their children. In the process, they end up creating people who are not satisfied with anything. The first step to answering this question then is to take a step back and examine how the tantrums come about, how you deal with them, and how you and your child feel throughout the process. By having empathy for your child and formulating a concrete plan to deal with tantrums, your child will know what to expect, and you will know what to do.

2. When it comes to playing, my son prefers dolls and girl clothes to cars and men's clothing. Is there a problem with that?
Playing is a fantasy and is the way to unload in the imaginary world what they cannot do in real life. Although boys may end up playing with a doll, this is nothing more than the exercise of care. You should celebrate your child's sense of caring, just as you would a little girl.

3. My son likes to play, pretend that he kills people. For a long time, I avoided buying toy weapons, but he turns any object into a revolver. Should I stick to the ban?
People often confuse the fantasy world and reality. Although your problem is common, if you feel it is becoming too real, then go with your gut. Since your child is interested in the weapons, playing new games that involve them is a great way to become more comfortable. Guns can be used for chasing bad guys, shooting water to win a prize, popping bubbles, or shooting aliens with lasers. Think like a child, and the possibilities are endless!

4. My son is very shy. He is ashamed to play with other children. How can I encourage him to interact with others?
Being introspective, quieter, having few friends, is not a problem, but a temperament, and is a part of the personality. Extraversion can also be a source of distress. Parents should only worry if the child cannot relate, participate in collective games, or

dislikes being with other people. In that case, you must seek the help of a professional. If you feel your child could use a little push, you can try and get other children involved with his interests. For example, bring several match cars to the park and see if other children would like to race them down the slide with him, or bring chalk and bubbles.

5. Sometimes I blackmail to convince my son to take a shower or change clothes. Am I acting correctly?
Bathing, brushing teeth, sitting at the table to eat, and taking vaccines are mandatory. But by the age of two, for example, the child begins to claim possession over his own body. One suggestion for when he or she does not want to bathe is to play the game of self-help, giving tools and negotiating: you buy a nice sponge, a special soap and let them wash with your supervision.

6. When I go out with my son, he always asks me to buy something (a toy, for example). If I do not buy it, he throws a tantrum. How should I act?
At 2 years of age, the child believes that everything is his. Then the parents take him to a lovely place, like a toy store. Put yourself in the place of the little one and imagine yourself in a place with everything that you like without being able to take anything. To avoid a scene, it is recommended talking to the little one before leaving the house and determining if there will be new acquisitions.

7. When I go out to dinner, my son does not sit quietly at the table. He runs around the restaurant and bothers everyone. Should I rebuke him?
You should most definitely not allow this to continue. Though all children have different energy levels, it is disrespectful and rude to allow your kids to run around. The toddler years are important for growing social skills, and you set the standard. Interact with your child at the table. Bring playdough and crayons, play 'I Spy,' and talk about things that interest them. As they grow, they will learn to entertain themselves healthily because you put the time into building their self-esteem.

The Only Child And The Arrival Of The Younger Sibling

You love your children the same way, but do your little ones think the same thing? The impact of the arrival of a younger sibling in the family is intense for the parents but especially for the children. Girls tend to identify with mothers, while boys tend to be more reserved. They will touch the mother's abdomen and agree to hear the baby's heart. They get excited about becoming the older brother or sister, but then comes the sudden split of your attention. Preparing your child for the arrival of your new baby is certainly worthwhile.

Before the baby is born, you can set up your nursery and allow the firstborn to get to know the new routine. Get a doll and show your child what it will be like to change, feed, and rock the baby. Practice being quiet and gentle. Though your child will not be able to care for the new baby, he/she can continue caring for the doll, as well as helping you by getting things that you need.

Though this newfound sense of responsibility is useful in building self-esteem, your older child is still just that – a child. Setting up a spot for you and the older child is a wonderful practice since there will be times that he/she needs your attention. It could be as simple as a chair that you two sit on to talk, a blanket for only you two, or a reading corner. Allowing your child to feel in control of their relationship with you can help deter from regressive behaviors developing, due to the new baby. Remember to positive reinforcement by complimenting your child on how well he/she is doing as an older sibling. Tell them how much you enjoy having a big boy or girl around!

Children Having Trouble Sleeping

Children need at least eight hours of sleep. Children are different in their sleeping habits, but all toddlers enjoy having a routine. Bath time is one of the best ways to get your child ready for bed. If your schedule doesn't allow for that, then you can look into reading a set number of books or watching a quiet cartoon. Some children benefit from a favorite stuffed animal or blanket. These things are comforting and can make a child feel safe. If the problem is staying asleep, you may want to look into a sound machine. There are so many light/sound machines on the market that you're sure to find one that suits your taste.

As your child grows, they are bound to have different excuses for not wanting to go to bed on time. Nightmares are a common occurrence in little ones and extremely frightening to deal with in the beginning. Take the time to explain that they are not real and teach them how to handle it on their own. Talking about something that made them happy that day, every night can double as their special tool to calm them if a nightmare occurs.

Above all else, if you want your household to enjoy restful sleep, establish ground rules, and stick to them.

The Sexuality Of Children

It is in the age range of five years that the child reaches a stage of development in which it differs as the figure of the man as the father, and the figure of the female the woman similar to the mother and understands the ties of relations of the outside world. However, even when the child already has a clear idea of female and male genders, it still raises doubts about their sexual identity.

At first, children will move according to the world, at home or in society, in a spontaneous way. It is only when parents or others express their idea that they are doing something that is not right that the child will suddenly or gradually perceive a conflict between their inclinations and the way adults expect them to behave.

Allowing children to explore their interests freely permits them to become who they want to be, sexuality aside. Pressuring a child to like certain gender-specific toys or mannerisms may have the opposite effect, and can lead to frustration.

Divorce: How Children Handle The Separation Of Parents

A divorce causes suffering and, in many cases, long-term problems for the children, whether psychological or social. This is because, no matter how much the couple believes in conveying harmony to their children, they are more likely to perceive conflicts.

Ideally, a couple who are divorcing should be able to maintain some degree of friendship that can make their lives less traumatic. Good sense and simple human respect are helpful. However, in the vast majority of cases, these qualities are ignored by one partner or both, which can start an irrational battle. The best solution: "Seek a psychotherapist, therapist, or marriage counselor to find a middle ground and a place to communicate well".

5 Psychology Tips to Understand Child Behavior

A child that cries non-stop cannot sleep alone, does not get along with his classmates at school is a child who could have behavioral problems. These characteristics in children worry parents, however, those are typical child behaviors. Children have a way of communicating by crying, expressing their aggression and fears with behaviors that may seem like mischief.

Let's take a look at 5 tips recommended by psychologists to handle some of these behavior issues, without having to despair or be aggressive with children.

1. Constant Crying

Children crying is often seen as tantrums or stubbornness. But that depends on the age of your child. When a child is less than 2 years old, crying is a way to communicate something that is not going well.

At this stage, a child cries because some physical or emotional aspect is causing discomfort. So it's good to look for a doctor or specialist rather than ignoring or trying to correct him or her. The tantrum phase and manipulation by crying usually begin after two years of age.

After age two, you'll need to be patient and have an understanding of your child's feelings. Having good communication and compassion can go a long way in changing their behavior.

2. Difficulties In Sleeping

Does your child delay sleep, even if he/she had a tiring day? Does he usually watch TV to try to sleep? If the answer is "yes," then it may be that the use of this device interferes with the quality of the child's sleep. This is because the luminosity emitted by television hinders the release of the hormone melatonin that is important for sleep. If your child watches a scary movie that intrigues or frightens him, it can cause his mind to stay awake and be anxious. Replace TV and movies with a book. Read to your child and discover the importance of this habit.

3. Fear Of Darkness

You put your child in bed, give him a goodnight kiss, and turn out the light of the room. Ready! That's where the crying and the fear of sleeping in the dark begins. This behavior is very natural.

At this stage, the child's behavior is guided by a very fertile imagination, able to create the famous monsters that attack the child while the lights are off.

Leave a low-intensity dim light or nightlight on in the room or adopt other methods such as talking more with the child, so she will be calmer. As time goes by, your child will realize that those monsters do not exist.

4. Aggressiveness

Does your child tease or hit other children? Or siblings even? This childish behavior must be viewed with care. Aggressiveness is part of our psyche; for it not to have major consequences, it must be worked on early.

When your child hits someone, talk to him. Ask him why he did it. It is crucial that a child learn to reflect and express his anger using words.

5. Fear Of Strangers

You need to work, so you put your child in a daycare that you trust. But he cries a lot and does not want to stay there at all. This type of behavior is normal because the child still has a very close relationship and is dependent on the parents. Hence there is the fear of abandonment.

In this case, you can spend time with your child at the daycare center, introducing the teacher and colleagues until he feels more confident. Then explain to your child that you need to go to work and that you will leave him with someone you know.

You can also leave your child with uncles, aunts, and grandparents. He will feel more secure and improve the bonds of affection with his relatives.

Chapter 2: Encouraging Good Toddler Behavior

One of the most effective ways to encourage positive behavior in children is through praise. Children seek love and recognition for their efforts and progress. Praise increases children's self-confidence and motivation by making them feel happy. It is important to give them confidence in their abilities and to show them that they feel proud when they behave correctly, thereby encouraging good behavior. Here are some highly effective tips to help encourage positive behavior.

Encourage Effort
Use praise to encourage effort and to enhance the progress of your child. A child who can use the bathroom alone for the first time or perform a task that he was not able to do before deserves recognition. In this way, it is encouraging the child's development and autonomy.

Reinforce Attitudes
Enjoy instilling some values that you consider fundamental, important, and positive. By praising and reinforcing attitudes, you help to develop social skills that will make relationships easier in the future.

Praise the Effort, Regardless of the Result
The effort must be praised even if the goal is not fully achieved. If your child did not receive an excellent grade, but studied and worked for this to be possible, it is important to recognize him. Praise is key to staying motivated and therefore improving your bottom line.

Praise Good Behavior
It is important to praise good behavior; do not save compliments only for great achievements. Small behavior improvements should also be valued. If we only pay attention at times where behavior needs work, children will feel inclined to do wrong.

Approve or Disregard Attitudes and Not the Child
As much as you consider your child to be very handsome, intelligent, etc., avoid telling him this often. This type of label turns out to be as harmful as the opposite ("you're dumb," "you're bad," etc.). Try to mark your approval or disapproval regarding attitudes, not the child.

Value the Achievements of the Family
It is important to value the achievements and efforts of the family. If a brother has conquered something, it is important to praise him, as well, the achievements of the father or mother. It is

important to recognize the effort of all the elements and celebrate the achievements in the family.

Rewards

You can also choose to reward your child, such as a gift, a trip to the movies, or candy if you want to reinforce an attitude. But do not make it a routine, because this can lead to only good behavior when rewarded. Most behavior should be rewarded only by praise. Also, you may be tempted to use the allowance as a reward. We do not recommend it. Never use the allowance to "buy" your child.

Rewarding the child for good behavior teaches them to understand that there is a direct link between action and consequence.

Remember that as a parent you are a role model for your children. It is essential that you be a good role model by providing them with appropriate rules and standards to follow. Consistency is the key. Children learn by observing others, and they will learn these qualities. With a little persuasion and positive reinforcement, you can teach, encourage, and create positive behavior in children.

How To Stimulate Good Behavior In Children

Educating our children was not easy. So I went after tips on how to encourage good behavior in children without having to punish and scold every second.

Stimulating good behavior in children is one of the best ways to impose limits, without having to apply punishments constantly. The only problem is how to do that. In most cases, our little ones tested our limits and seem to do anything not to obey.

Here are ways to stimulate good behavior:

Be The Example

Being an example is the most effective way we have to teach our children anything - both good and bad. When it comes to encouraging good behavior in children, it is no different. Here are a few examples of what you can do for your child to learn.

Catch your child's attention when you split snacks with your husband or when you have to wait in the bank queue, pointing out that adults also have to share and wait too.

Realize The Good Behavior

If you are like any parent in the world when your child is behaving well, you leave him playing alone and take advantage of the time to do anything you may need to. But when your child is behaving badly, you direct all your attention to him to resolve the situation. Your attention is what kids most want, so to get this attention sometimes children will behave badly. The best way to encourage good behavior in children is to pay attention when they are behaving well and to take your attention from them when they are behaving badly. This is completely counter-intuitive for us and can be a difficult habit to cultivate. But once you get used to it, it will become easier and easier.

A great way to do this is to play with your child when he is quiet in his corner and praise him when he obeys you the first time you speak.

Understand The Stage Of Development

This tip is easy to understand. Each child has a behavior; however, you cannot require a child of three to act as the same as a child who is ten. That is, do not try to go to a three-hour lunch with your little boy hoping he will be quiet for the whole lunch. Do not want a two-year-old child not to put everything in his mouth. Each age has a phase, and it is no use wanting to demand different behavior from a child.

Have Appropriate Expectations

This is a continuation of the above tip. Parents have high expectations. This is not wrong when expectations are possible. For example, do not expect a tired child to behave well, or a one-month-old baby to sleep through the night.

Create Structure and Routine

A child with a structured routine tends to behave better. They already know what to expect and are used to it. A child with a routine feels safe and thus lives more calmly. A child without a routine has a sense of insecurity that will disrupt much in the time to educate and encourage good behavior.

Uses Disciplinary Strategies

Rather than humiliating or beating children, there are positive disciplinary strategies that teach, set boundaries, and encourage good behavior in children. Some of these are: give options, put somewhere to think, talk, give affection and a system of rewards (reward can be a simple compliment, it does not have to be gifts or food).

Understand That The Bad Behavior Worked So Far

If throwing tantrums and disobeying worked for him to get your attention so far, changing this behavior will take time. He will have to realize and understand that you will no longer pay attention to him when he behaves badly, but when he behaves well.

Instilling good behavior practices in young children is a must for any responsible parent, but sometimes it can also be quite complicated and laborious. However, beginning to instill this type of behavior as early as possible will help build a good foundation for the child's behavior and attitudes in the future. It is necessary to be aware that in the first years of life the children are like "sponges" and results will be better if you begin to show them early and direct them to appropriate behaviors of life in society.

Here are some more ideas to help parents with the task of encouraging good behavior in their children.

Models To Follow

Children tend to mirror the behaviors of parents and those with whom they coexist more closely. Therefore, be careful about your behaviors and language used when the child is around to avoid misunderstanding ideas and misconceptions about how you should behave towards others. This includes talking properly and behaving politely to both your partner and family, as well as to the child. Try to avoid loud, unstructured arguments when the child is around. We do not mean you can't disagree with your spouse, because the child must also be aware that these exist. But try to have the arguments always controlled and civil around children.

Be Firm

Parents should be affectionate, but still adamant about instilling discipline in their children. It is important that the child knows how to respect his parents, even when he does not have what he wants. Understanding when to say "no" at the right times is an important step in your education.

Positive Body Language

Your body language has a huge impact when you are trying to instill a particular behavior in children. Given the height of the child, a parent standing while correcting the errors and applying discipline is often viewed as authoritative. It is advisable to place yourself at the same level as the child's eyes. Sit next to the child while talking to them and always maintain eye contact.

Establishing Limits

It is fundamental to establish limits, rules, and consequences for unwanted behavior. Increase limits on children to be able to distinguish right from wrong. They need to know what is not acceptable and clear reasons that make it wrong so that there is no doubt in the child's mind about the behavior to adopt.

You started tracking your child's progress long before he left the warmth of your belly: in the tenth week, the heart began beating; on the 24th week, his hearing developed and listened to your voice; in the 30th week, he began to prepare for childbirth. Now that he or she is in your arms, you're still eager to keep up with all the signs of your little one's development and worries that he might be left behind. Nonsense! Excessive worry will not help at all, so take your foot off the accelerator and enjoy each phase. Your child will realize all the fundamental achievements of maturity. He will learn to walk, talk, potty, and when you least expect it, you will be riding a bicycle alone (and no training wheels!). He will do all only in his time.

Stop taking developmental milestones so seriously. For example, your 7-month-old son will be able to sit alone and at age 3 will be able to ride a tricycle. Consider what is expected for each age just for reference. The best thing to do is to set aside the checklist of the abilities your child needs to develop and play together a lot. There is no better way to connect with and develop your child than through playtime.

To help you even further in realizing the goals mentioned above or processes, I would like to mention some tips here that stimulate a child's intellectual, motor, social, and emotional development:

Rainbow

The baby starts noticing colors at around 3 months of age when the vision is no longer so blurry. That is why, at this age, the idea is to stimulate with strong colors, which can be in toys or mobile in the crib. Babies also love contrast: you can see that stripes are not missing in children's toys. At about a year and a half, your child will begin to notice the difference between one color and another, even if he does not know the color's name. So, start saying: "Let's play with that blue ball" or "Take the red tomato from the salad." This way colors become part of their day to day life.

Books

The role of parents is fundamental for children to learn to love reading and to make books a pleasure, rather than an obligation. According to the latest edition of the Portraits of Reading survey in Brazil, for 43% of readers, the mother was the main influence for developing the desire for reading, and for 17%, the father was the one who played the role. From the third month of your child's life, you can use plastic books in the bath. From the sixth, when the baby can already carry objects to the mouth with his hands, leave cloth books in the cradle - in addition to being able to bite them, he will not be able to rip the pages! At all ages, talk about the cover, the pictures, the colors and let the child turn the pages.

Memory

Memory is a form of storing knowledge and must be permeated by a context. Start by helping your child memorize words by showing a represented object. If you are walking on the street and crossing a bicycle, point and say, "Look, son, a bicycle." This is how he will build associations. From the first year, he will say a few words and try to repeat the names of what you show. But it is from the age of 2 that the ability to retain information increases.

Creating

Create characters and a dream of fantastic worlds. All of this is important in developing the creativity of little ones; it also contributes to problem-solving. To make the narrative more exciting, how about testing the improvisational ability of the two of you? Separate figures from objects, landscapes, colors, foods, and animals – they can be drawn or cut from magazines. While one narrates, the other can select images that portray elements that should be included in the narrative. The challenge is to be able to fit them together so that the narrative continues to make sense. By age 7, as the child is already literate, you can help him record your adventures in small booklets.

Always Ask

When picking up your child from school, you say, "How was your day?" And he says, "Cool." It was not exactly what you wanted to hear, right? To avoid generic responses, develop the questions so that the child needs to express what he thinks and justify his response. Ask: "What did you enjoy most today?" And he will be forced to develop more elaborate reasoning, requiring him to work linguistic and logical skills. At 3 years old, he can already relate experiences he went through and say whether those were good or bad. At 4, you can ask for details, descriptions, and names of colleagues who were with him.

Blessed Doubt

"Why does a dog not eat pizza?" "Was Grandma Ever a Child?" Although child questioning can make adults uncomfortable or embarrassed, these are essential for understanding the child's world. It is the process of distinguishing between real and imaginary (which occurs around the age of 4) and the construction of relations between known elements. That's why the "why questions" are so important in the child's development process. Even if you do not know how to respond to everything your child asks, show that his or her concern is relevant, and recognize when you do not know the answer.

Play, Clean, Play

As your child plays, insist that he engage in one game at a time, to build concentration. "Do you not want to play bowling anymore?" From age 2, your child can help clean up the toy he was using, before picking up a new one, so he also develops the sense of organization.

Belly-Down

Your child begins to strengthen the body between the first and the sixth month. Because thick motor development (involving the activities of large muscles such as sitting and walking) occurs in the head to toe direction, the first step is to strengthen the neck muscles. Beginning the first month, give your child at least two periods a day supported belly downtime on a flat and firm surface. In this way, the baby can lean securely and lift his head. At 6 months, he will start to sit alone. Arrange several cushions around him to help him get stronger.

Clap, Clap, Tum, Tum

One of the best ways to develop motor coordination is to teach rhythm to your child. To do this, just use your hands. From the seventh month, clap with him to the sounds of your favorite songs, interspersing slow songs with other accelerated songs, so he can see the difference. You will see that your baby will be able to hit his little hands.

Everything Fits

From the age of 7 months, the baby begins to hold objects; in about a year and a half, he will begin to put pieces together. Besides being a good exercise for coordination, the child will learn which part will fit within the other. For your child to enjoy and learn from this, he can play with pots and plastic mugs while you prepare lunch. From the age of two and a half, also offer small puzzles (about six pieces).

Step By Step

Climbing stairs is a great exercise to develop agility and coarse motor coordination, as well as assisting to strengthen muscles. At 1 year of age, the child can already perform the activity, but only by placing both feet on the same step, one at a time. With growth, he will gain strength and balance until by age 3, he will probably rise by placing one foot on each step alternately. Even at this stage, it is important that he be accompanied by an adult to avoid accidents.

Bonding & Trust

Establishing relationships of trust is important for the development of the child. The first people he does it with are the parents. For this, one factor is essential: never lie. If the child goes to the doctor to take a vaccine, do not even think about saying that you are just going for a walk. If he asks if the injection will hurt, be honest and say it will, yes, but it will pass. The experts are all in agreement: explain everything. Tell him he's going to get wet, it's going to hurt, he's going to be cold, so he knows what to expect and learns to trust what you say.

Congratulate your child when he is good at something, encouraging him to continue. If scolding is necessary, pay close attention to how to do it. Saying "what you did was naughty" is quite different from saying "you are naughty!" Do not let the child think that the criticized trait is part of his personality, so he will not incorporate this trait into his self-image.

Chapter 3: Behavior Management Tips & Tools

We've made a list of tips that will help you deal with issues that influence children's behavior.

1 - Fights can be difficult for a child. It's even worse if this conflict happened between the parents. Understand the importance of maintaining a harmonious home where feelings are accepted and discussed without judgment. Disregarding a situation that has been recognized by your child, can be harmful to their emotional development. If your child understands an argument or feels the tension in your home, explain that yes, his feelings are valid but that he is safe and loved.

2 - Letting your child make decisions and letting him dream about the future without fear will help him be a happier and more confident child. Allow self-expression and applaud your child's desires. Reinforce and "I can do it!" attitude.

3 - Getting your child to know, appreciate, and respect other cultures is not only a cool thing to do, it can help them in the future. Understanding other ways of living will allow them to be more approachable and respectful, allowing for better relationships and success.

4 - Helping your child to feel loved and special, in addition to his siblings, can shape his identity and present him with a healthy sense of self-esteem in the present and future. Everyone needs to believe in themselves!

5 - Children lie and do not always understand the gravity of a lie. Understanding where they are in development is necessary here. Talking about what harm lies can cause is essential in developing their grasp on how all the world works.

6 - Teaching gratitude to your child creates a happier child and can be fun. People love good news, especially children. What's better than having something to be grateful for? Teach your children to be grateful for the small things such as the weather, their toys and clothes, the fun they have at the park, or even the hug they receive. There will always be something to be grateful for, and this way of thinking can change their world for the better.

7 - Humor is very important in the individual and social development of your child. Laughing is healthy. Being able to see the humor in situations can help build personality.

8 - Children are surrounded by issues that can cause anxiety and fear. Fear of the unknown is fear of most everything for young children, not to mention the size difference for a child in an adult world. Explore with your child and teach them to feel capable and safe.

9 - You may have heard about "The Terrible Two's". Be aware of what to expect from the tantrum phase. Most parents would agree that the terrible two's is referring to 2 and 3-year-olds. Remember to practice patience and understanding. Children at this stage are ready to communicate and get around on their own, and we need to convey to them that they are still learning. Make learning fun by giving them jobs as a helper with tasks you would normally do alone.

10 - Each of a child's actions has a meaning, but it is not always clear what it means. Pay close attention to the context of your child's behaviors, and you will understand what each behavior of your child means.

11 - This may seem like nothing to you, but for your child, it can mean a lot: Respect your child's growing emotional skills. Their knowledge of the world is rapidly expanding and can become overwhelming. Never embarrass a child for feeling a certain way.

12 - It is normal for some children to feel uncomfortable in new situations. Giving them the rundown before you leave the house allows them to know what to expect and it can help with confidence.

Be Aware Of The Difficulties Of The Child

According to experts, persistent difficulties in performing tasks can indicate signs of hearing problems, vision or hyperactivity, and should be analyzed before raising the conclusion.

Certain behaviors may direct parents to find out if the child suffers from these disorders. It's important to pay attention to troubles your child may have and discuss them with your doctor regularly. All children develop differently, so don't jump to conclusions on your own.

Behavior Modification Techniques

The great number of learning studies carried out in the behavioral field (especially by B. F. Skinner on) allowed the delineation of an intervention methodology named *Applied Behavior Analysis (ABA)* and *behavior modification.* This technical-scientific approach aim to preventing, managing and solving children's behavioral problems. In this context, "behavior" refers to actions and abilities.

Below, I will explain to you the main evaluation strategies and educational intervention. Specifically, I will specifically focus on:
- procedures for proper observation of children's abilities and difficulties (behavioral assessment).

- I will focus on strategies to enhance positive behaviors and on strategies to decrease problematic behavior.

Skills And Behavior Assessment

- Consider the level of development of the child a precise evaluation of his abilities both in the cognitive and behavioral field. To help you: download the free developmental checklist at the beginning of this book.
- Consider the strength and weak points of your child to organize suitable learning situations.
- A functional assessment aimed at understanding the motivations behind the behaviors. Check if there were any changes in the child's family life (for example, the birth of a brother), or if your child has slept enough and is in good health. Sometimes challenging behavior is the first sign to indicate that the child is not well.

Teaching Skills To Children: Strategies

As already stated, behavioral management involves educational work aimed at acquiring and consolidating various functional skills and competences. The main strategies used to acquire and consolidating skills and abilities in children are:

- Prompting and fading
- Modeling
- Shaping
- Chaining
- Reinforcement

Prompting And Fading

The technique is to provide the child with one or more stimuli in the form of instructions (Prompts), to achieve the desired skill. Prompts are usually obvious and are proposed at the exact moment the performance should occur. These can be divided into:

- Verbal suggestions
- Gestural indications
- Physical guidance

Depending on your child's level, they can be provided in the form of vocal verbal instructions (such as explaining, telling, etc.) and non-verbal (such as written, images, etc.). These prompts must necessarily be reduced or modified (Fading) to allow the definitive integration of the ability in the behavioral repertoire of your child.

Modeling

Much of our learning is based on imitation. Much of what we have learned in our lives, we have learned from observing other people. In these cases, other people are the model for our behavior. The ability to imitate is, therefore, a requirement of great importance for human beings. The modeling technique consists in the proposal of learning experiences through the observation of the behavior of the subject that acts as a model.

The modeling technique is used when a parent intends to teach his child, through imitation, certain new behavior that he is unable to implement quickly through other modalities. This is a technique that allows reaching important goals at the level of behavior, but, above all at the relational level. It allows, in fact, to adapt the adult's expectations to achievable goals, avoiding making negative feelings on the child such as frustration, and establishing a virtuous spiral of reciprocal reinforcements: the adult reinforces the child for small improvements and such improvements reinforce the adult in return.

Shaping

In practice, with this technique, we will repeatedly reinforce those behaviors that, although far from the targeted behavior, progressively approach the goal.

B.F. Skinner describes shaping with the analogy, operant conditioning is compared to a ceramist who shapes a piece of clay. The ceramist's product will have a specific shape but we will not be able to find the precise moment in which this form will appear. Likewise, is a certain response from a child is not something that appears suddenly but the result of an ongoing process of formation.

Reinforcement must, therefore, be provided initially to behaviors that are relatively easy for the subject, and then reinforce those that are increasingly closer to the target behavior. To do this we need to break down the final objective into small sub-goals. In this way, we will reduce the expectation of the child. Gently pushing to his small improvements every time, until reaching the final goal.

Chaining

Chaining or step by step is a strategy used for teaching complex skills. When teaching complex skills such as personal autonomy like dressing, washing hands, brushing teeth, you need to split the tasks into small, separate steps to facilitate learning. When you use chaining, the first step is to prepare and complete a task analysis, identifying all the smallest teachable units of behavior that constitute a behavioral chain.

Task analysis to teach your child how to brush his or her teeth might look like this:

- Take the toothbrush
- Squeeze a small amount of toothpaste onto the toothbrush
- Wet the toothbrush under the tap
- Brush the teeth

There are two procedures for teaching a chain of behaviors: forward chaining and backward chaining. Using forward chaining, the behavior is taught in its natural order. Every single phase of the sequence is taught and reinforced once the entire sequence is completed correctly. Using backward chaining, all behaviors identified in the activity analysis are initially completed by the adult, except for the final behavior of the chain. Then it is the turn of the second last step and so on. An advantage of backward chaining is that the child has the feeling of having successfully completed a task before mastering the entire procedure. This gives to him confidence and motivates him to continue his efforts.

Reinforcement

Reinforcement is the most important and widely applied principle of behavioral analysis and regulates most of our daily activities.
Reinforcement can be defined as a consequence that strengthens a given behavior with the chance that it happening again in the future.

Reinforcements can be of two different types: positive and negative. When it comes to behavior, positive and negative do not mean good or bad. They simply must be intended as algebraic signs that is the add and subtract. The positive reinforcement increases the probability that behavior is repeated thanks to the positive effect that this provides. For example, a child is learning to read, the mother is close to him and when the child reads correctly, she tells him: "good" (positive reinforcement); reading acquires a positive value for the child because for him it is a source of attention from the mother. Negative reinforcement also increases the probability that a behavior will be repeated because this removes a certain negative effect. For example, the child cries because she's hungry her mother rushes to feed her, in similar situations, when the child will be hungry, she will cry again to get her mother's attention. Negative reinforcement is not punishment. Punishment does not lead to the extinction of behavior but it will make it less likely to occur in the future.

In punishment, there is no learning. Certain behavior is inhibited, blocked (usually momentarily) without learning new behaviors. In reinforcement instead, both positive and negative, there is learning because in the case of positive reinforcement we learn a new behavior that has positive effects, in the case of negative reinforcement you learn a new behavior that is useful to stop something negative.

How to effectively use reinforcement when working to teach new behaviors?

- Reinforcements should be customized based on child preferences: observe the child's interests and motivation to determine which reinforcements are best.
- Reinforcement should be immediate: this means that the reinforcement should be delivered immediately after the desired behavior appears.
- Reinforcement must also be associated with behavior: in other words, the level of reinforcement must adapt to behavior.
- You associate tangible reinforcements to social reinforcements: sometimes it is important to combine praise with rewards.
- Continuous reinforcement and intermittent reinforcement: it is important to constantly decrease the number of reinforcements given over time.

Reinforcement is an important principle that determines an actual change in behavior. It is used in all ABA programs but it is also something that happens naturally in your everyday life. Think about your days and your life: you will realize that almost everything is driven by the principle of reinforcement and that all our behavior is encouraged or not by the response we get.
Below we will explain through simple examples four proven behaviors modification techniques.

Behavioral Intervention Techniques

Parent's behavioral intervention techniques are usually based on the consequences of a child's behavior. Those interventions attempt to change behavior through the application of positive or negative consequences. Positive and negative consequences increase or decrease the frequency, intensity and duration of a given behavior, they are used as rewards or sanctions.

When applied correctly, positive consequences can be very effective in modifying children's behavior. Experience suggests that whenever positive consequences are immediate, regular and modified in order to avoid a certain habit, children can reach good results. The first step that parents have to do to intervene with positive consequences, is to observe the child's actions in order to determine which consequences can be truly reinforcing for the child, that is, which prizes, situations or actions are effective to strengthen the desired behavior.

The use of negative consequences for the child can be carried out through some techniques including planned ignoring, the cost of answer and time-out. Since the negative consequences are effective regulators of human behavior, these must be applied adequately and safely in a controlled environment.

Time-Out

The time-out can be used in two ways. One of these is the typical reaction to unwanted behaviors: "go to your room for five minutes" or "sit for five minutes in punishment." This type of time-out will be seen by the child as a negative conclusion or punishment. Probably, the most effective approach is to think at time-out as a pause to the child's poor behavior and not as a punishment, a short period of time that allows the child and the parent to have a few minutes to distance themselves from negative behaviors, in order to process them and calm down.

What happens after the time-out is very important! Some believe that, after a time-out and before anything else, the child has to come back and apologize. Others instead conceive time-out as time spent moving away from negative behavior and then being able to rejoin the family without the embarrassment of having to apologize publicly. This second modality is preferable because it allows the child to reconnect more naturally to the activity interrupted and, on the other hand, avoids the emotional problems linked to having to apologize.

Cost Of Response

This technique is used to remove something pleasant from the child. In other words, fines or penalties will be applied when negative behavior occurs. We use the cost of response to avoid providing the child with feedback to inappropriate behavior in conjunction with positive rewards for appropriate ones. For example, if the child doesn't observe some previously established rules, this procedure involves the loss of a previously earned token or the failure to earn one in the future: "If you don't want to take the coat off the ground, I'll do it but you'll lose a token ".

Token Economy

The establishment of a Token system at home is quite simple. The basic idea is that a child earns tokens every time he achieves an established goal. If the child fails to reach the goal there are no negative consequences; tokens are in fact assigned only to the achievement of the goal or positive behavior. Once a token is earned, this can never be taken away. This allows the child to form a strong link with positive choices. In some cases, as previously mentioned, it is also possible to earn extra credits in order to further incentivize the child's motivation toward positive behaviors. For example, if the child helps to lay the table, as agreed, he earns a token; in addition, if he also offers himself to help to clear up, he could earn additional credit.

To create an effective Token Economy it is necessary to think carefully about the way the table is presented. This needs to contain the description of goals to achieve and relative rewards, also evaluate where to place it in order to make it visible.

Positive Communication

The way we choose to communicate is absolutely important. Rather than say "don't do this or that" we try to communicate our intent using descriptive and positive sentences. "Don't swear" could be expressed as "we use polite language" or "we speak to people respectfully"; "Don't hit" the same way, it could become "we use our hands gently". Try to contain comments and negative reactions. Our interventions, including Token Economy, will be less likely to succeed if we use a punitive tone of voice or aggressive body language. The child may change some of his behaviors for fear of being punished, but this will not help him to grow. Moreover, when the fear is no longer present, the child's behavior will again tend to worsen.

If the child behaves as we expected, reward him by identifying a precise moment and a place. For example, before going to the mall we could say: "If you sit calm and safe while driving, you will receive a reward of two tokens", or "if you sit politely at dinner, at the end of the meal you will get a cake". With these sentences, we have made an accurate and positive description. Always remember to describe the behavior you want.

Chapter 4: Crying & Tantrums

Why Toddlers have Tantrums?

Tantrums are a normal part of a child's development. It is a communication channel chosen by the child to communicate that they are upset or frustrated. Tantrums happen when kids are hungry, tired or uncomfortable; they aren't able to communicate and express what they feel, want or need. There is a neuro-psychological explanation for the tantrums of toddlers. The frontal regions of the brain that determine executive functions (our capacity for planning, self-control, and reasoning) mature later than the other areas of the brain. Thus, it's natural that, in many instances, children have tantrums, because they are not psychologically able to express themselves any other way. One of the most common tantrum reasons is that children cannot handle limits and have great difficulty hearing the word "no".

How To End The Tantrums Of Children?

Leo, now 6 years old, is the son of the publicist Shirley Hilgert, 39, author of the blog Macetes de Mãe. Shirley, who today is also the mother of Caetano, 3, says that when her oldest was 2 years old, there was a situation when he yelled the entire time she was at the cashier's area. While she was embarrassed by the situation, she took a deep breath and put herself in her son's shoes. "He wanted something he could not have; I squatted down and explained to him that he was not going to get it and why. I knew if I gave in at that moment, he would make the same outburst the next time. I stayed firm in the decision."Leo bellowed a little more at the store exit, but, as predicted by his mother, he never repeated the "show."

The Good Side Of The Tantrum (Yes, It Exists)

Does the tactic adopted by Shirley work for everyone? In other words, is there a formula to end the tantrum? The answer is: it depends on the child. A recent study by the universities of Amsterdam and Utrecht (Netherlands) in partnership with the universities of Cardiff and Oxford (UK), analyzed 156 surveys from 20 countries involving 15,000 families with children aged 2 to 10 years who had disruptive tantrums. The researchers detected two groups of techniques most used to deal with the problem: those based on behavior management (combined, for example) and relationship building (dialogue, among others). For children with more frequent disruptive behaviors, the study found that the most effective method is a mixture of the two strategies.

Tears Heal: Why It Is Important To Let Your Child Cry!

What makes empathy an essential point for dealing with so-called "children," especially for strengthening family ties? Within this approach, there are many ways to act. Child psychologist Mayra Gaiato, a master at experimental psychology and behavioral analysis at PUC-SP, suggests three steps: prevention, combined, space and support.

1. Prevention

That's right! For the specialist, parents should warn the child what will happen so that she can "prepare," especially in situations that precede something she does not like or does not want to do. Sometimes you can even use some instruments, like a timer. Does your child cry every time you announce it's time to go home from a party? Before that time, make it clear that you are leaving in five or ten minutes.

In addition, you need to make sure your child's needs, both basic and subtle, such as your feelings and desires. Often, children give indications (by action or facial expression) that he or she is unhappy, before the explosion. These signs may vary from one to the other, of course, but among the most common are: need of sleep, hunger, fatigue, increased aggressiveness, moodiness and impatience. For example, it is no use taking the little one for a walk when what they need is nap time. That will turn into crying for sure! Over time, it will become easier to identify these "triggers."

2. Combined

If the tantrum happens, even if the day is well planned, the second step is negotiation. If your child has a problem when it comes to sitting at the table, the idea in this situation is to lower to the child's height, maintain eye contact and make a combination, such as: Let's have dinner now, and you can play again soon after. "It does not mean giving in and explaining to the child why she cannot do what she wants," says Mayra. Do not confuse empathy with permissiveness.

3. Space and support

If the behavior continues or worsens, the specialist suggests, as a third and final step, that the adult waits for the child to calm down. "You have to wait, give her space and silence. Show her you're around, but cannot talk while she exhibits that behavior. Her brain will understand that she did not get what she wanted and that her "strategy" does not works. Then, when she is calmer, complete the process with "sensory support," as the specialist says, that would be a hug or a kiss, to help soothe the child.

Learning to deal with this behavior that is part of your child's development.

Space For Routine

A child needs routine, so he knows what to expect, and what he can and cannot do. This provides security, and it is the transmission of affection. This holds true for everyday situations such as bathing, dining, and going to school. For this to happen, the whole family needs to be organized. It is like confusing the child with the values of the family: can you imagine how chaotic a home in which right and wrong mix? To keep the rules, it is also essential to make it easier for them to be fulfilled: if you want them to always behave in a public place, they will not let you sit in a crowded restaurant or wait for them to calm down in a bank queue.

Value The No

You already know the importance of saying 'no' for your child to learn to mature and realize that you will not have everything at hand when they ask for something. "Children who are never contradicted end up becoming angry, aggressive, and unhappy adults. After all, the world will not always give an unconditional "yes" if parents have always said that to their child," explains the Child Psychoanalyst Anne Lise Scappaticci. The little word "no" should not be wasted in completely unnecessary situations. When used without moderation, the word "no" can lose strength and invite disobedience.

Act On Punishment

It is of no use to punish children under 2 years of age. They are not mature enough to realize that they have done something wrong. For example, if your child throws a toy on the floor or against someone and you take the toy, that's a punishment for her. When the child is older, it is worth removing something important for the child, like the classic "No TV". Punishments, when properly applied, serve the sense of justice that all children have. The lack of punishment, on the contrary, disorientates them. A quiet, serious look at a child is a particularly effective kind of punishment. The purpose of punishment is to make the child think.

To be educative, the child needs to understand the relationship between what he did and the consequence. The punishment must happen at the same time because children have an immediate vision: they have not yet learned to think in the long run. That is, after some time, they do not know why they are being punished, they forgot the original offense.

We are not talking about spanking, pinching or slapping. That is unnecessary.

Tantrums usually occur around the age of two, which is when children leave the baby stage and gradually begin to perceive themselves as an individual with their own opinions. Children at this age, due to the lack of maturity, express themselves through the tantrum to show their desires and feelings.

How You Deal With The Tantrums

Children learn much by examples. The best way is to have self-control during small tantrums. If we deal with the tantrums of children with aggression or punishment, they will learn that aggression is acceptable. It is important for parents to control their own feelings when their child gets out of control.

The biggest mistake that parents do at the time of tantrums is to do the will of the child to prevent him from continuing to scream or cry. Although unpleasant and embarrassing in many situations, do not give in.

When parents make a decision, and they go back as a result of the child's tantrum, the child will begin to understand that one can always make a temper tantrum and at some point, the parents will give in.

But Then, What To Do?

At this point, I should stress the importance of parents helping their children deal with frustration. Only this will grow strong and fearless adults.

Of the many demands that exist when tending to children, the difficulty they have in dealing with the "no" is undoubtedly the greatest. These are children who grow up with great difficulty tolerating frustration. They do not know how to cope with that emotion. They do not know how to accept it. And, above all, they despair! Imposing limits, lovingly, is the best way.

What Do Mothers Have To Say?
Who has not had a situation when their child had public tantrums? Here is an excerpt from the words of a mother facing some similar issues. "In these last months, he has been very silly and stupid when he hears to 'no' from us. He crouches on the floor, cries, sometimes hit us, or beats himself (in the head). At dawn, for example, if I do not breastfeed at the time he wants, he screams a lot, kicks me and does not listen to me at all," explains the mother.

She knows that this phase is complicated, requires patience and lots of conversation, but sometimes the situation is beyond her control. "I often lose my temper and talk a bit louder, but it's not the right way to deal with it. Sometimes I ignore or try to distract him with other things, like toys, drawings, painting. I think it's just a phase that is known as "Terrible Two's," which many mothers go through during this same age group."

Positive Discipline

Let's take another example to understand: Dandara Brito (mother), 27, João Miguel's(child), now 2 years and 3 months old. Dandara began to use positive discipline at home, a pedagogical approach based on mutual respect and cooperation, which aims to help parents in their child's education.

Positive discipline is considered a compromise between the rigid and permissive way of educating the little ones, giving them limits, but wherever possible, with choices. It is a program based on the studies of two Austrian psychologists, Alfred Adler, and Rudolf Dreikurs, from the beginning of the last century.

Positive discipline (a way of educating that has been gaining more and more acceptance), aims to encourage children and adolescents to become responsible, respectful, resilient and provides resources to solve problems throughout life.

"João's tantrums began to happen at 1 year and 8 months. Usually, it occurs when he wants to do something not allowed or when he has a tiring day. He screams a lot, cries; sometimes he throws himself on the floor, "she explains.

Dandara points out that she seeks to validate her son's feelings and understand what he wants to convey at that moment.

"It's a phase where they are maturing their emotions and usually cannot deal with them. I always try to search, and the best way I can handle these moments without being permissive but being kind. And I try to apply positive discipline and non-violent education", she says.

Around the age of two, the parents are faced with a child full of desire and ready to open the shout when being contradicted. There are days when he only eats food if it is on the plate. In others, they do not want to eat. Hence, he asks to watch TV or use the iPad, but at bedtime. And when he hears "no" from his parents, he starts beating and throwing toys, cries desperately and throws himself on the floor. Later, he is reluctant to enter the bath, and when he enters, he is reluctant to leave.

Such situations become routine in the lives of parents of children approaching two years of age when the phase dubbed "babies' adolescence" begins.

And, behold, these parents, who were getting used to a baby who accepted almost everything passively, are surprised by a child full of will and ready to scream when being contradicted. The good news is that this is not only normal but a crucial part of child development. And learning from child experiences at that age will help shape the way he deals with his feelings in adulthood. The second good news is that there are many clever ways to deal with these behaviors as long as parents are armed with strategies and patience.

BBC News talked to four child behavior experts to learn about the importance of this phase around the age of 2 to 4 years in development and raised ten practical tips to guide parents in day-to-day situations.

What Happens Around The Age Of Two?

"It's a phase where the child makes incredible discoveries and gains tremendous ability to interact, but the areas of self-regulation in his brain have not yet developed," explains Ross Thompson, a professor in the Department of Psychology at the University of California, Davis and president of council of the organization Zero to Three, dedicated to this age group.

"The most important thing is for parents to understand that this child is simply unable to control their emotions. This understanding will help them see it more constructively, rather than think it is challenging their authority. Telling a child to calm down will not work at this age. It is up to the adult to help her put her feelings into words and manage them. "

"The child begins to realize that it is not an extension of the parents, but a person with desires. And to these new desires there is intense frustration, accompanied by cries and cries," says educator parental Elisama Santos.

Children at this age are dying to use their newfound autonomy. This maturation of emotional control in the brain lasts until the early 20s, but the most critical phase of this "babyhood" usually goes away by 4 years, when children increase their repertoire to express themselves and understand the world. Until then, if parents get carried away by anger and become punitive, situations tend to get out of control. If instead they act calmly, empathically, and offer strategies for this child, this one will learn tools to deal with their emotions - something that will help them through adulthood.

When The Child Strikes

When contradicted, many children from a year and a half, beat up on parents or caregivers. Unable to express their frustration in words or to calm down on their own, they resort to physical reactions. "stop beating, you're grounded!" - The child will become more nervous and will not know what to do with their feelings. Instead, explain to the child what he is feeling and giving tools for him to overflow. "I know you're upset, but we do not eat sweets at this time of day." "When you're sad, hit this drum rather than beating people," or "bite this toy instead of biting Mom, "for example.

Repeating this several times, the tendency is for the child to begin to understand their feelings and the resources to manage them. A hug helps calm down in tantrum moments.

Elisama Santos gives similar tips: teach the child to clap or roar like a lion when they need to release the energy of anger.

"I also suggest talking in a tone of curiosity: 'Did you see that your little hand hit me? You're the boss of the little hand, you take care of it.'"

"This is difficult in a culture that blames parents when kids are making tantrums," she says. "(But) remember that your child is not purposely trying to humiliate you - he simply cannot handle the situation. Your job is not to punish him, but to empathize, validate his emotions, guide him, and keep him safe. Let people think what they want. "

Help the child express in words what she is feeling (frustration, anger, irritation) and offer her arms and arms - even if she does not say, 'Mom is here when you want a hug.' And let her cry, making sure she's in a safe space if she's floundering.

Changing the environment, looking at the sky, taking a turn, and taking the focus off the tantrum motif often helps to "turn off the pump." But experiencing the sadness of frustration is part of the (difficult) process of growing up. Cure heals and is a tool to calm down. Learning to recognize feelings and deal with frustration is a process that begins at this age.

The Limits

Keeping calm does not mean giving in to the child's desires, which would give her a counterproductive message: hereupon "if I make a tantrum, I will get what I want." If you give in, you will not strengthen the muscle of resilience or teach the child to deal with frustration, something essential for adulthood. The way is not to be permissive, to say 'no' when necessary and to welcome the frustration that comes from that.

Children are testing their power and their choices, and if the father does not stick to the limit he has set, the behavior will continue, and it is necessary to impose time limits on the TV or tablets. If the child does not want to put on his seat belt, put it on, be impassive, and move on. He will gradually realize that even if he does not cooperate, the belt will be put on anyway.

Do Not See Acts As Manipulation

For children so small and in times of stress, little use is made of asking "why did you knock?" or start big discussions - they are too small to understand, and the tendency is only to increase tantrums. Children are provocative; they will say, 'I hate you,' they will beat you. If we see this as manipulation - while they are typical behaviors of that age - we still tend to react angrily.

Providing A Chance For The Child To Choose

To prevent long-lasting battles and the child from taking control of the family routine - at meals, at the time of dressing, when leaving, give acceptable choices to children, who are dying to exercise their newfound autonomy. The trick is always to give two choices to children and set limits. For example, in the case of toys scattered around the floor of the house, you have two great ones: If you do not clean up, Mom or Dad will have to spend time doing it, so we'll not have a book to read at bedtime.

The idea is to give consequences to the choices of the children, but appropriate to the situation.

Instead Of 'No,' Positive Reinforcement

To Elishama Santos, children of this age say "no" to (almost) everything because they are used to hearing a lot of "no's" from parents - who, although well-intentioned to protect children, can use a more efficient strategy: positive reinforcement.

It's no use saying that she should not put her hand in the socket, because what she's going to fix is just the socket. It's better to give instructions on what she should do rather than what she shouldn't.

Playing More - Choosing Battles

Turning everyday activities into jokes helps relieve stress in boring tasks, says the parent educator. If you use a robot voice or make tinsel to wear or brush children's teeth, it will take that phase more lightly and easily. Avoid getting into all the (exhausting) battles with children. If it does not interfere with the functioning of the family and does not hurt anyone, I recommend leaving it there - for example, if your child decides to leave the house with a shirt that does not fit with the pants.

Plan To Prevent Tantrum

Identify patterns of behavior to prevent tantrums: for example, changing the bath or bath time. And if you know what caused the tantrum of the previous day, you can try to stop it today with conversations. 'Remember that yesterday was a very difficult time for bathing?'.

Is 'Educational' Slap Going To Help?

Experts advised by BBC News - whether to teach limits or to get the child out of dangerous situations - will not help the educational process so crucial at this stage. Violence tends to make children angrier and more challenging, and parents more punitive - in a vicious cycle. The same goes for verbal assaults. The child will only find that it is not loved enough - and it is very bad to spend this phase of life finding it.

Lost control? It has salvation

Sometimes the parents themselves get carried away by the situation, even if they do not want to see each other screaming or losing their patience with their children. It may be a great time to teach children to take responsibility for their actions.

If the situation allows, it is also possible to "take a break" by saying 'Mom will take a moment to think' this is a possible way out. It gives you a moment to breathe and to elaborate on what choices you will offer your children. And parents can benefit from having another adult around whom they can turn to when they are about to lose their temper - and ask them to take the lead. Finally, experts point out that the tips given above will have to be repeated a few times until they are internalized by such small children. That is, prepare your patience.

In the beginning, it takes time and effort for parents to manage their own reactions. But the payoff is huge: it will come in the form of more self-control of children, more cooperation in daily tasks and more positive cycles of interaction.

Chapter 5: Common Behavior Concerns

As they grow, all children are likely to go through challenging situations that cause worrisome thoughts. The role of parents is not necessarily to eliminate anxiety but to help control it. Prothero, a psychologist who specializes in childhood anxiety disorders, said that regardless of whether a child was diagnosed with anxiety or not, the way parents can help does not change. "We have seen many children referred for treatment in the last five years, and this seems to be increasing," the therapist told The Huffington Post UK. Parents can really do a lot at home to help a child who is suffering from anxiety.

If you notice that your child suffers from anxiety, you can be sure that you are not alone. Parents should only worry if they notice that their child's anxiety is having a significant effect on school or their relationships. Many children do not know what they feel when they are anxious, and this can be very scary and oppressive.

Identifying Signs of Anxiety in Your Child

I'll mention some examples where a mother connected the dots of some of the problems their child was suffering from, for example: bed-time problems, with the potential anxiety they might be suffering from through open, polite conversations and understanding.

"My son is almost 8 years old, and the first time I noticed his anxiety he was 4 1/2 years old," said Jordan Martin, 35, whose son is anxious before going to school. "I had to take him to school despite signs of anxiety, which were unusual [in his personality]: crying, shaking and holding his belly," said the mother. "I would drop him off at school and cry when I got home... It was very important to be consistent for him to go to school, but I felt terrible."

Martin cited as other signs of anxiety the child's fear of bed-time; he said that "bad things" could happen. "He cared about silly things like his school backpack not being at home, anything related to change," he added.

Salma Shah, whose 5-year-old daughter has anxious thoughts, often said that the behavior has been constant since she was a baby. "As a baby, I remember her turning her back on all the other babies and turning to me, distracting me by pointing at things," Shah explained.

"One of the main symptoms I noticed when she grew up was her attachment. If she had a 'playdate,' she would always be by my side and never spoke voluntarily to people, not even to family members with whom she had always had contact. "

Natasha Jones, 35, said the anxiety of Ella, her 7-year-old daughter, came when she was saddened to think about illness and death in the family. This was reinforced the first time she saw Harry Potter and Cinderella. The films sparked concern about death and the possibility of losing parents. "She was constantly worried if she was alone at home or with another family member," Jones explained. "The problem got worse if I was not at home. It affected her concentration on things like homework or playing, and she became very sensitive before bed, with frequent stomach pain. "

Now, how to help control a child's anxiety?

1. Divide Situations Into Small Portions

When a child is feeling anxious about a scenario, it is tempting to help her avoid it. But with that, he will never develop confidence. Instead, help them break up the situation they are having trouble with into small pieces and make lots of compliments with rewards as they tackle each 'piece' before moving to the next level.

For example, if a child is socially anxious, encourage him to attend small meetings and allow him to get used to it before attempting a slightly larger party.

2. Use Relaxation Techniques

Martin creates a "safe place" for the son, where he can feel protected and calm before going to bed. She talks to him using relaxation techniques, such as a soft tone and positive phrases.

The words parents can say during this relaxation should be the most appropriate for the child's needs. I use the first person, which works well, for example: 'Repeat in your mind:' I'm safe, I'm home wherever I am, it's okay.' A soft tone, with a light touch on the shoulder or chest, works well. And Martin is a great example of the same.

Be careful not to use negative words, so instead of saying, 'Do not be scared,' say something like: 'You're safe, all is calm, and all is well.'

3. Teach Breathing Techniques

Breathing, in general, helps anyone who is feeling anxious to draw attention to the action of breathing and not to the cause of worry. Controlling this can create a sense of calm and prevent future anxiety attacks. Martin said he uses these techniques to calm his son. "I use the technique of inhaling through the nose counting to four and then exhaling through the nose counting to four," he said.

The goal is for children to regain control over their emotions; so if they face a 'scary' or 'uncomfortable' situation, they can resort to safe and effective strategies, such as the powers of a superhero.

4. Stimulate A 'Happy Thought'

Martin says he tries to tell his son a statement positive every night before he goes to sleep and every morning before he goes to school - which is when he feels more anxious. "He now asks for this specifically," he said. "I think he feels safe and supported, knowing he can focus on this when he goes to sleep or on the way to school. My husband was the one who started with the 'happy thought.' My son asks, 'What is my happy thought?' ".

Encourage the children to choose their own happy memory because it is their mind, and only they can know what animates their spirit.

5. Prepare For Anxiety-Provoking Situations

"We have come to places or parties early, so my daughter has not to walk among a lot of people, "Shah said, explaining that the daughter feels anxious in social situations. She said that preparing for possible anxiety situations in advance allows the daughter to deal better with them. "She responds kindly to kindness," she added. "We also highly commend her when she actually attends a party or event to reinforce her achievement."

6. Over time, Expose Your Child to Different Circumstances

Shah said parents should never worry about the possible embarrassment of the child being "too attached." They should focus more on building trust in their children. Do not push them too hard. But kindly, over time, expose them to different circumstances that will get them out of their comfort zone.

7. Do Not Get Angry, Work As A Team

"We try to be understanding and recognize my daughter's problems," explained Jones. "We've done a lot of research to try out techniques that would suit Ella, and one of the best ways to reassure her is to talk to her. Telling her that she's not alone and that other children have the same fears, including me, is comforting. We work as a team, and she knows it will take time for her fear to go away".

8. Create A 'Book Of Worries'

To help children with long-term anxiety, you can create a" worries book," and through that, you can encourage them to see what things make them anxious - their triggers. Just in case they are old enough to do this, have them write their thoughts in a 'book of worries.' Jones said the daughter uses this technique, writing her thoughts into a "box of worries."

9. Talk To Other Parents

For parents who do not know how to help their children deal with anxiety or anxious thoughts, talking with other parents to know their techniques can give ideas. Sometimes the solution is closer than we think.

10. Seek Professional Help If Anxiety Persists

If anxiety does not improve over two or three months or is significantly affecting your child's ability to socialize or go to school, you must seek professional help. Therapists who specialize in children can be consulted privately or through their GP. For example, the British government recommends that children with social anxiety have 8-12 sessions of cognitive-behavioral therapy.

Children are anxious by nature. In the car, they ask every five minutes how much time is left to complete the trip. At school, they may experience belly pain on test days. At home, they hang around the kitchen until dinner is served. The willingness to anticipate situations and the excitement of what is to come is part of child development - but to a limit. When they start to generate suffering and get in the way of everyday life, it can be a sign of a bigger problem.

According to the American Association of Anxiety Disorders, between 9% and 15% of the population aged five to 16 suffers from the disorder, which is characterized by a set of physical reactions, psychological and behavioral that precede a real or imaginary situation.

Carolina Schneider Silva, a psychologist at the Santo Antônio Children's Hospital of Santa Casa de Misericórdia in Porto Alegre, explains that anxiety attacks are disproportionate reactions of children to the stimulus they receive, whatever they will be. In Julia's case, a single line served as a trigger.

Crises can be characterized by a sense of fear and apprehension, marked by a period of tension or discomfort in the face of some event considered dangerous, even if it does not offer real risk. When exaggerated, they may appear in the form of tachycardia, muscle tension, tremors, shortness of breath, fainting, and bowel problems.

Know the Signs, Treatments and Know What to Do

The symptoms of an anxiety disorder may arise suddenly or gradually. Possibly, so they go unnoticed by many parents.

External Stimuli

Childhood is a period of many changes, and the degree of anxiety goes through oscillations as the child grows. Whether at the beginning of the school year, in routine changes or changes in the family environment, external stimuli generate new sensations and emotions.

In this age group, there are two types of anxiety disorder most common: Generalized Anxiety Disorder (GAD) and Anxiety and Separation Disorder (ASD). Science cannot yet explain why some children develop the problem, but some factors seem fundamental:

- The development of anxiety disorders results from the interaction of multiple factors such as genetic inheritance, the temperament the psychiatrist Gustavo Teixeira, a member of the American Academy of Psychiatry for Childhood and Adolescence and author of books on the same subject.

Experts argue that the picture is also linked to the excess of stimuli that children currently receive. They are subjected to greater social and emotional pressure from both the family and the school, for example.

- It is necessary to know the children and to be alert to changes, be they physical or behavioral. The most common ways of expressing anxiety are through recurring concerns and difficult to control. Together, there may be restlessness, easy tiredness, difficulty concentrating, irritability, and trouble sleeping or staying asleep.

How To Deal With Behavior Disorder In School?

A school brings together students from completely different personalities. There are those quieter students, the more introspective, the communicators, and those who never obey the rules. In the latter case, delivering an activity in the classroom can be quite an exercise in patience. However, you need to be cautious with children because behavioral disorders are much more complex than a simple tantrum.

Early childhood education should be ready to welcome children in general, but it is true that the most questioning, for example, presents a challenge for the educator. When you are faced with a student who has such characteristics, the best way is to be able to deal with each particularity brought to the school environment.

What Are These Behaviors?

Conduct can be diverse and range from challenging questions to physical aggression in extreme cases. However, it is important to point out other behaviors that are related to the disorder referred to in this article: rule violation, disobedience in the classroom, bullying of the child to other colleagues and teachers; cries, impulsive actions, provocations, discussions, and school dropouts.

Preparation

No doubt, there are many parents and teachers who are not prepared to deal with such situations. However, warning children energetically is not a step to be taken, although many do. That's because the little ones can feel challenged and insist on the attitude that motivated the warning made.

How To Deal Then?

The common point of all ways of dealing with behavioral disorders is dialogue. It is important always to establish communication between the child and the adult. Ask the child, the reason for such disobedience and try to have the confidence of the little one. Of course, this is not so simple, but there are ways to reduce the causes of these behaviors:

- Family therapy: support groups that work to develop the relationship between parents and children are a great alternative. In this situation, experts advise parents to establish effective communication with the child and to show them the limits to be placed on the child's behavior.

- Psychological follow-up: the child who presents some behavioral disorder in school can also find ways to improve their relationship and interaction with the environments in which they are. Psychological counseling can mean a very good way for the little one, from the moment therapy can help you get along with everyone around you.

- Multidisciplinary team: nothing more indicated than to act together with a diversified team, that brings together therapists and school teachers in the search for the improvement of the child's behavior.

And The Parents?

Parents and guardians should establish a satisfactory communication with the pedagogical and therapeutic group in order to arrive at an adequate response to the disorder presented.

It is very important that everyone has patience with the child since the child must find trust and authority in adults. To act cautiously does not mean ceasing to impose limits. On the contrary, the limits are indispensable. Adequate follow-up and parental attention are important determinants of behavior disorder.

Chapter 6: Friends & Siblings

Can small children be friends? They can but in their own way. That means you should be prepared to see one bite the other, take the toy without asking ... These are things of the age that need to be understood. In the range of 1 to 3 years, the child is still egocentric, and the question of the possession of objects is very present. Therefore, it is common for them to take a toy from the other's hand and walk.

The little ones are in the famous oral phase, in which they use the mouth as a means of discovering the world. As long as they do not know how to talk, they end up sometimes hitting for no reason, just to get what they want. Of course, if aggressive behavior is too frequent and intense, it requires parental attention. It is not necessary to deprive the one who was caught up in the other's life but to ensure that it happens in the most protected way possible, supervising and separating in case of aggression.

Not infrequently, a more passive child becomes friends with a bossy one. The experts consulted say that the leaderships of the group begin to dawn with 4 or 5 years. When this happens, others become his followers - and make no mistake about their little age: the leader realizes the strength his opinion has over others.

When the teacher identifies this in school, he should use strategies and jokes to dilute this configuration so that roles are reversed in some situations: followers become leaders, and the leader becomes a follower - this can also be done at home by parents. If conflicts arise from the relationship between a leader and a follower, it is recommended that each child should orally expose the other to how he felt and what he did not like. They should listen and try to resolve the situation with each other.

Shy Children

More introverted and shy children may have difficulty making friends. In such cases, parents may approach a class in the playground of the building, for example, and introduce the child, asking if he can play with them. So, next time, he will already have a reference on how to act. You can also invite classmates to attend your home. That way, they will have what to talk about in the room, plus memories of fun times together.

But if the child is never called to any party and seems to be always isolated, the ideal is to do a job with the school to detect why this happens. You can also enroll your child in extracurricular theatre or sports classes that help decrease inhibition. Just do not press it.

If your child is very sociable and makes friends easily, rest easy. Just be aware of whether your child is not acting that way to get attention and can do a little more work with a concentration in the classroom. Point it out that there is time for everything.

Friends – Siblings

Who said siblings could not be good friends? In these cases, one only needs attention if the youngest becomes a" shadow "of the brother and ends up having no personality. Well, then, talk about the importance of having your own attitudes.

There are also cases where siblings have no affinity. Parents should be aware of the context in which the lack of friendship happens and the expectation they have of that relationship. In general, siblings will be friends but often go through situations of jealousy and competition. It may also be that they have different interests, which seems like a lack of friendship, but is related to gender and age. Parents need to look at how they relate to the family (mother, father, and siblings) in order to identify whether they have a strong or superficial bond because the child perceives and tends to have similar behaviors.

Leaving

If the parents look back, they'll remember that some of their own friends walked away for a while and then came back. You have to stay calm and keep in mind that this is a process of building the bond of the child. Another feeling that can arise in such a situation is jealousy. When there is some dependence on friendship, attention is needed. If we identify something negative, that does not benefit both parties. It is necessary to stimulate new friends. The adult should show that the child can discover affinities with several children.

Outside The Party

Make no mistake, this will happen sooner or later, either for financial reasons (it's expensive to invite all the students) or affinity. In these situations, the adult needs to be prepared to face the frustration - of the child and parent. Parents must accept that it is not the end of the world and explain that some people identify more with each other than with others.

The opportunity is ideal for sitting with the child and asking why he thought he was so close to the birthday boy. Sometimes he thinks he's friends with the other, but he's not reciprocated. It is important to have this understanding, that some people give the impression that they are our friends, but they are not.

Colorful Friendship

From the age of 4, children begin to perceive each other better, start comparisons, and have a greater perception of their own body. It is common for situations to arise from one wanting to kiss and embrace the other. Some even talk about dating. This is largely a reflection of what they see daily in the media, that is, an imitation of behavior. When faced with such issues, parents should teach the child that he is able to express affection in various ways - with words, drawings, and jokes together - and to say that he should not kiss another person on the mouth.

My son never wants to leave his friend's house. What to do?

Parents should keep in mind that no matter how friendly they may be, there is no way to force the bond between children. The identity that made them be friends does not necessarily happen among their children. And adults should be prepared even to get upset. If this is your case, it is best to avoid contact between children, especially when there are no others to interact separately. Prefer to date only with adult friends.

The Friend Is a Terror

One way or another you will come across those friends who are a "terror": they make a mess, they mess around the house, they speak profanity ... The desire to berate the colleague can be enormous. If it is to your child that the message must be given, explain that there are several ways to behave and that the way the other acts do not please you, pointing out how the line has been crossed. The same must be done with swearing. In general, small children do not know what they mean, but if they realize that it causes anxiety in their parents, they can repeat it on purpose, just to manipulate them, just like the tantrum. Therefore, be very calm in explaining that this is not acceptable to say.

Away From Home

Generally, it is at about 4 years that the child starts to go to friends' houses and, from 5, can be prepared to sleep outside the home. Knowing the routine and habits of other families is positive, as it broadens the worldview. It is inevitable, however, that the child will make comparisons and question aspects such as "in so-and-so's house I could stay up late. It is a good chance to teach your child that each family has its own rules - which are not better or worse, just different.

It can happen the opposite also: your son sleeps there and discovers that he does not identify with the style of the family (schedule, food, fear of a pet). Listen and see what he has to say and do not force him back. One option to keep the friendship is to take walks with the colleague elsewhere or let your child visit you for short periods of time.

My Idol

It is common for children to choose a friend as an idol for a while and want to have the same clothes and toys or to repeat their attitudes. Over time, they realize that they do not have to copy the colleague to have their friendship and stop it. But it is good to be alert when this behavior is exaggerated, asking, for example, why the child wants an object or is doing it. Explain that friendship does not depend on it. If it does not work, seek help from a psychologist. At the other end, the "copied" child can tell his friend, "Be yourself."

Is There Anything Better Than A Long-Standing Friendship?

So that your child does not lose contact with the friends of the first school, you can invest in pajama nights, movie sessions, walks, and activities in which they maintain their coexistence. It's wonderful to keep childhood friends. When there is a story, something special has happened. If a healthy friendship perpetuates itself, it is because it continues to have something to add.

He Said Goodbye

It is evident that friends will leave your child's life for one reason or another. One example is if a friend should move away. This can generate in him an even greater sadness than the simple exchange of school. But how to deal with loss does not change. There are children who suffer less and others, more. This is a frustration that needs to be managed.

You can talk to your child by welcoming him and legitimizing his feelings, without neglecting this pain, at the risk of him becoming even more distressed. At the same time, it is important to encourage him to find resources to face this situation, either by making new friends - by fostering encounters with other children - by maintaining contact with the friend who moved. Through social networks, for example, it is easy to establish video or text conversations among children, even though they live in different countries. They can also be encouraged to send letters, emails, pictures, and drawings to each other.

Beach Friendship

The holidays are fun and pass by fast. Therefore, they are usually so intense for the child. When she makes a good friend on the trip and shares pleasant moments with him, it can be painful to say goodbye. Here, the same tips apply when the friend changes a school or a city. Explain that there are moments of farewell in life, but that it is possible to keep in touch. It may be that the feeling of loss still lasts a few months, but the child has the power to reorganize very quickly.

We all want our children to behave well. In fact, most of us would dare to say that we want our children to be friends with each other. Unfortunately, parents who dream of their children playing together as they grow up usually feel more like judges who never take vacations.

Although we are still trying to figure out how things work with three children, we had our first two children seven years ago. They get on very well. Part of that is personality, and another part of it is because we try to intentionally create an environment where they would grow up and naturally become friends.

Here are some tips I and more importantly, we, as a community, have learned to cultivate friendship between siblings:

1. Give Them Space

Our nine-year-old son needs some time alone. He needs silence and needs rest because of his older brother's role. Even if you do not do this every day, we've talked to him since he became a brother, and whenever he wants, he can spend time alone in his room.

We respect and protect that time, which often means keeping younger siblings away from his room. By being introverted, I understand his need to be alone and in silence to rest. Our two young children do not need time alone, and that's not a problem. But by respecting Will's needs, we're helping them understand that people have different needs. This will help Will to remain patient with his brother and sister, and will also give the two younger ones time to play together. We also never forced them to play together. We respect their literal and figurative space.

2. Do Not Force Them To Share

At least not everything. We think sharing is a lot easier when you do not have to share everything. Let the children have at least some toys or books that are only for each of them. They can share these things when and if they want to. They cannot go into each other's rooms and mess up what is not theirs without permission. Being a child is already too difficult. Having personal properties makes things a little easier. This is also a great way to teach boundaries.

3. Form a Team

No, you do not have to have enough children to form a team literally. But you can promote a teamwork environment within your family. When we do something together, even if it's something small like cleaning the car (okay, that's usually a big task) or something even bigger like finishing a long walk when we all wanted to give up, we celebrated our teamwork. This also applies to the way we talk to them when they are away from us. They know that they must always be united because they are a team.

4. Limit The Time With Friends

We value the friendships they have, but at these ages, most of the time with friends is during class time or at baseball practice. When they play at home, sometimes they are together with a friend, but usually, they play together. And they like it. Because the time of watching TV is limited, their imagination is free to explore while they build memories together.

5. Stop Judging

Unless your children are about to hurt each other, try not to interfere. If we constantly control their quarrels, we will be teaching them that we do not trust them to be able to resolve by themselves. And no matter what we say, each of them will probably feel like we're taking sides.

Problem-solving is a very valuable skill, but your child will not have a chance to learn if you volunteer to do it for him all the time. And believe me, we know it's tempting, even if it's just to get some quiet time.

6. Invest Quality Time for Each of Your Children

Even though this seems like one more way to build the parent-child relationship, and it really is, it's also a great way to combat sibling rivalry. When the children's love reserve is full, they are much less likely to compete for parental attention. Because they already have it.

Sibling rivalry is normal and cannot be completely eliminated, but I'm not even sure if it should be. Even if listening to your fighting kids drives you crazy, you know they are learning valuable skills that they will use for the rest of their lives. Our first interactions with other people in life are usually with siblings. It's a great way to teach our kids to relate to others, solve problems, and be kind when they do not want to be kind. These are just some of the ways we help our children be friends with each other.

Chapter 7: Discipline

Nowadays, the question of limits and punishments seems to be in everybody's head. Parents are always looking for ways to discipline their children that are fair and effective, so they do not feel guilty for traumatizing the little ones. We quickly learn that our children grow up and that getting punished and other methods of discipline that work on younger children have little or no effect on older children. After all, sending a teenager to sit at a designated time-independent location will not work for its purpose.

As children grow effective punishment requires a whole new approach. An effective measure to discipline older children is to remove the privileges they enjoy. Like, for example, taking a cell phone, iPod, television, or video game. But it is important to be sure that punishment fits the "crime." For example, do not arbitrarily take your phone and give it back when you feel like it. Just as with time, any punishment you put in place should have limits and set rules in order to be effective. Punishment should be proportional to failure, and it is always desirable that they are combined in advance.

A minor infraction should result in the removal of a privilege for a relatively short period of time. Save the most serious punishments for times when your child really does something wrong. In addition, it is always good to explain to the child why you chose such an attitude to punish him, and exactly what you expect from your child in order to have their privileges again.

Lack of discipline hinders learning, professional performance, and even prevents people from reaching their goals in life. Therefore, it is important to learn to be disciplined. As children, we are able to understand routines established by society, and this is good for both group-living and personal fulfillment. Each activity has date, place and time to happen. The task is to be done at home.

The child needs pre-established routines to develop discipline. They need to know clearly what to do, when, how, and what we expect from them in each situation. Many children who seek the cerebral gymnastics course have difficulty learning and have poor results in school. In many cases, it is noted that this is a consequence of a lack of discipline.

To help these children improve their behavior, sometimes parents and schools develop pre-scripted lessons to be given to the child. This eases anxiety and helps a lot. Children pay more attention and carry out activities successfully.

Games Help Develop Discipline

There are examples where schools have developed various kinds of infographics to explain to the child what is expected of him in each activity to be developed. One of the classroom activities that most encourages discipline in the age group of 6 to 10 years is the pedagogical games, which teach the student to obey rules, respect the rights and limits of others and organize the space used for the plays.

Discipline is something that comes from home, but if the child still does not have it, the school needs to give him the necessary stimulus. Here, I would really like to reinforce that discipline contributes incredibly to concentration, reasoning, creativity, memory, self-esteem, and the health of the mind.

How Can Parents Contribute?

Many parents stay at work all day and resent leaving their children at home with no activities to do. There's no television. So the greatest tip of the pedagogue is to create a daily agenda with the tasks that children must do after school.
Write down on a paper the activity and time that the task should be completed. Vary activities each day. You have to be a bit methodical with the child. Leave a clear and objective list with bath time, television, homework, and jokes. Create a

study routine, teach him how to organize room space. Organization is very important.

Another good tip is to set aside time for free activities. The little ones are going to adopt this!

Are days when your little angel looks more like a little devil?

Here are some good practices for educating and disciplining your child which have been gathered from across viewpoints, training and curriculums:

Educating and disciplining children implies, among other things, establishing clear rules and limits. This is not always easy, even more so these days, but if parents adopt positive educational practices early on, it is possible to prevent future difficulties and problems. Cláudia Madeira Pereira, a clinical and health psychologist with a doctorate in clinical psychology, points out some good practices that will make this task easier:

1. Talk To Your Child

Even if you are exhausted after a day at work, take some time out of your day to talk to your child. At dinner or before going to bed, ask him how his day was, using phrases such as "Tell me what you did today," "Tell me about the good things that happened today" or "Did something bad happen?"

If your child is having a bad day, he can resort to several solutions. First, allow him to speak and listen to him without judgment or criticism. If you prefer, look for positive aspects that you can highlight and praise. Also, tell him about "what" and "how" to better deal with similar situations in the future.

2. Pay Attention To Good Behavior

Sometimes children learn that bad behavior is the best way to get parental attention ... This is especially true for children whose parents pay attention to them only when they misbehave, even if that attention is negative, scolding them and rebuking them.

In order for your child to see that the best way to get their attention is through good behavior, praise him / her and / or offer affectionate gestures (giving him kisses and hugs) whenever he does or even tries to do something good, such as helping set the table or doing a message, for example.

3. Promote Your Child's Autonomy And Responsibility

Some tasks, such as dressing in the morning, can be difficult for children. Even though it would be quicker for you to dress your child, you would prefer to encourage their autonomy and responsibility. Help your child by giving short and simple instructions on how to do the tasks.

To do this, use expressions such as "Take off your pajamas," "Now put on your shirt" or "Finally, put on your pants." Finish with a compliment, using phrases like "All right, you did a good job!" Sometimes it will not be enough to tell your child what to do; you may need to show him "what" and "how" to do it.

4. Establish Clear Rules

Be clear with your child about a set of rules. First, explain the rule succinctly and concretely. Second, make sure your child understands the rule and knows what is expected of him. In order for your child to be able to respect the rules more easily, try to give clear and simple directions, empathically and positively.

Phrases like "It's time to go to bed. Let's go to the room now, and then I'll read you a story," usually work. It is common for children to challenge the rules in the early days but stay firm and consistent. Repeat as many times as necessary so that your child realizes that the new rule is to be followed.

5. Set Limits

When you need to correct your child's behavior, try to be patient, and stand firm. Tell your child that a certain behavior must stop, explain the reasons, and inform him of the consequences of not obeying. In that case, preferably use phrases like "If you keep doing, then ...". Immediately and consistently implement the consequences whenever bad behavior occurs.

But do not resort to punishment or physical punishment (such as beating), as they only aggravate children's behavioral problems. Prefer to take a hobby or an object appreciated by your child for some time.

6. Stop The Tantrums

Although it is not easy, try to ignore the tantrums, not paying attention to the child at such times, as long as there is no danger to the child, of course! If possible, step back and pay attention to it only when the tantrums stop, so that your child realizes that they can only get their attention when they stop throwing tantrums. At that point, prepare yourself, because your child will put him to the test.

At first, it is normal for tantrums to get worse. However, by systematically applying this method, the tantrums will eventually disappear. Remember that what you want with this is that your child learns that tantrums are no longer a good way to get what you want and that the best way to get the attention of parents is to behave well.

To achieve this, you must be aware of your child's good behavior and value these behaviors whenever they occur, for example, by giving a compliment, a kiss, or a hug. If you do, the child will feel more accompanied.

7. Learn to Control Your Negative Feelings

There are times when any mother or father feels the nerves at the edge of the skin. When this happens, there are several ways you can act. First, make sure that your child is in a safe place (such as a crib or room), then withdraw for a moment to calm down. Then try to do something to help him or her. You can, for example, listen to some music or take a few minutes of meditation. When you feel calmer, go back to your child and start again, using conciliatory phrasing in a sweet tone, like "I felt I did not know what to do, but I do know what to do with it now."

8. Have (A Lot Of) Patience

When you raise your child's communication (verbal and non-verbal) empathic and positive, will be contributing to a healthier and happier relationship between both. Educating and disciplining your child will require a great deal of your time and patience. No wonder they say being a mom and dad is tough, but at the end of the day, it will be well worth it because it is the most rewarding job you can have.

Chapter 8: Connecting

The day to day work is always very hectic. Parents do not stop for a second. I think that everyone who has a child lives the same tiresome routine and always looks for the best way to connect with their child, although this is not always easy. Take care of children, clean the house, organize tasks, and I know that many mothers and fathers find themselves alone in these tasks. They are really like an octopus because they have to deal with a thousand and a few things in a single moment.

With all this upheaval, we can put aside the connection with our children, letting stress overwhelm us. It's easier to leave our kids a little time, maybe two, in front of the TV. Phew, this time gives us a lot of things: sweeping, bathing, tidying up, storing clothes ... The problem is when it becomes a routine, and little by little, it seems easier for us to silence our children by giving them a thousand and one toy so that we have a desired moment of peace.

What we do not tell ourselves is that this moment of peace can cost us dearly. In the end, the disconnection with our children will make us parents ruder, that to get the son to do what he wants, he should scream, curse, threaten, and even beat.

Following some advice can help us to establish an effective connection with our children on a daily basis:

- No cell phone when you are with the child.
- Turn off the television
- Make at least one activity together a day.
- Ask how your day was, listen to it calmly.
- Play
- Observe their behavior.
- Set priorities
- Exclusive time when you are with the child
- Tell him how you feel. Ask him how he feels
- Read stories together

Remember: THE BIGGEST PRESENT YOU CAN give is the best way for you to connect with your child.

Not to complicate things, but if there are simple and effective ways to connect with your child, why not use them? How about opening up space for something like Positive Discipline?

Now, touching upon the topic of positive discipline, we learn to focus on empowering our children so they can become able in solving their problems on their own. We also recognize that physical and psychological punishment are not resources that foster children who are autonomous, responsible, and independent.

I have noticed the frustration of some mothers when they come across a public place with their children and ask themselves: "Am I the only one experiencing these tantrums and moments of desperation? "I see such" nice "children! At this moment, the best thing to do is to be empathetic and very careful in attacking you and your children. You should prefer keeping the connection with children than thinking only of pure discipline. When we keep our attention focused on them, it helps to improve the relationship and achieve success in the strategies we employ.

There is no way we can connect with children without devoting quality time to them. It is not enough for five minutes at breakfast or five minutes before bed. Being wholehearted with children requires us to be willing and "some" time of exclusivity - parents and children - mother and child or other similar combination by combination stress: connection, time, love, dedication, and clarity of family attitudes and agreements.

We are always overwhelmed with everyday tasks. We cannot let life pass like a steamroller over us. How many times have you looked throughout the day for your child and really felt connected to him? Want a better connection than a bear hug, an eye on the eye, and a surprise kiss? Children are not our possessions - they belong to themselves. So we need to hear what's on their minds. What they dream, what they expect from us as parents and their fears. Have you listened to your child carefully?

Think in terms of quality rather than quantity. I'm not referring to being stuck or in the presence of the child 24 hours a day. On the other hand, being at home and not having time for a valued connection is not functional. Being there is simply very different from being connected. If you are doubtful if the time you are dedicating to your child is of quality, ask yourself the following questions: "Have had moments throughout the day where I am really body and soul with my child?" "Have I hugged and told my child that I loved him often enough?"

We are upset or disappointed when our children exhibit inappropriate behavior. We cannot forget that children are immature, and as such, still cannot deal with emotions. Anger, frustration, or sadness may trigger the red button. So we need to remind ourselves that we are the relievers and the blueprint for our children, and most of the time we have to play the 'middle field.' The next time your child goes off the hook or behaves inappropriately, avoid any outbursts of violence and seek more effective solutions. Violent shouts do not educate, but frighten, humiliate, and reduce the child's connection with his caretaker.

Access your power of compassion! We are less tolerant of children than of most adults we live with. Children are still in the process of developing and learning - they need compassion much more than our criticism. The way we respond or react to a particular behavior of our child may mark him for the rest of his life.

Avoid excluding and promoting the connection. When your child does not seem to listen to you or even be aggressive towards another child, it is the moment that he or she needs you most. We have a tendency to reprimand and punish. Avoid doing this - show acceptance and at the right time, talk about what happened. Otherwise, the message you will be passing on to your child is that you only validate it when he is "nice." Remember, there are no perfect parents or perfect kids. We are human, and mistakes are good ways of learning.

Try to see your children as timely teachers. Children are able to awaken the best and the worst in us. In the worst moments, where we feel a lot of anger, our tendency is to go to the attack and punish in several ways: beat, scream, or other forms of punishment. However, instead of pressing children to be our ideals, we can adjust our anxiety or expectations and learn to direct our attention to our own feelings and how to deal with them in the best possible way. We are parents with a strong desire to be right. So we can use our experience as lessons. We can learn to see the world through a childish gaze. In this way, we will learn to be less critical, pessimistic, and punitive.

Be more curious. We tend, as adults, to think we know all the time. Our son will tell us a story and we anticipate counting the end (at least in thought). What we do not know is the size that this story has for our children. Children feel the need to be seen through our curious and loving gaze. So ask more about the characters in the story, get interested in the plot, laugh, be amazed, vibrate, and fantasize along with your child. Just be curious.

What to do for dinner? Who's going to pick up the kids at school today? And if it gets cold, are they well wrapped? There are so many decisions that parents have to take every moment that they often forget to take breaks to enjoy the company of the little ones. It so happens that, in parallel with caring, these moments are also responsible for creating strong and lasting bonds - which is fundamental to your child's cognitive and emotional development early on.

"Children who have strong ties to their parents have greater learning capacity and are better related to each other," says pediatrician Cid Pinheiro, of São Luiz Morumbi Hospital (SP). A survey published this year in Finland proves this. By accompanying 700 families over seven years (from the baby's birth until he entered school), scientists were able to observe that in those children and parents who had healthy relationships, children were more likely to learn to regulate their own emotions.

Another important point is that in these moments of complicity, you get to know much more about your child, their likes, desires, and what he thinks about the world around him. You will be surprised and proud. This exchange is one of many that strengthens the bond with your child. Here are 11 tips to put into practice!

1. Create Family Traditions

Children, especially younger ones, feel safer in well-defined routines. Use this to your advantage, including connecting times with your child throughout the day's activities. For example, sing a song at bath time, serve breakfast in the form of smiling faces (with bread, pancakes, fruit) and even pause together to meditate and relax.

2. Enroll In A Course With The Child

Music, arts or swimming lessons can be a lot more fun with the children on the side, so much so that there are nowadays several establishments that offer courses aimed at children and parents. Prepare to be delighted to witness each new achievement of your child, such as mastering a new step or increasing your breath to stay underwater and see you happy to be able to share it first-hand with you. The partnership in these moments of discovery and learning will make them closer.

3. Take A Different Walk

Who does not remember a sunny morning at the beach or a lazy afternoon fishing with the whole family? Many memories are lost in adulthood, but special moments surrounded by people we love always remain. Even though the effective memories of this phase are not accessible to consciousness, they are still present. Use creativity when deciding the program! It does not have to be anything elaborate, as long as it fades from the routine. A day at the amusement park, a visit to the museum, a picnic in the square ...

4. Read To (And With) Your Child

The tip is basic, but it counts a lot! It is worth, first of all, to create a special climate for the time of reading, whether it is a corner with cushions on the floor or a half-light. Try to interpret the story by giving a different voice to each character to stimulate the imagination. For example: if the character is more thoughtful, speak slowly, and tone down. If he is tense, use a firm voice. And have your child read to you later or make up some story. Besides being a delight to hold while reading, the books are an invitation to the curious questions of the small and almost inexhaustible subject for future conversations.

5. Build a Camp in the Room

Kids love an adventure, and you do not even have to leave the house to fulfill that desire. Put pillows and cushions on the floor and build an improvised tent with the sheets. It's time to disconnect all the electronics and act like you're in a real camp. Connect a flashlight in the dark, tell stories, and enjoy sleeping together. They will not forget that night so soon!

6. Stipulate The Day Of "Today You Can!"

The routine with children is full of rules and schedules, as it has to be. But a little flexibility does well, as well! Did he ask for popcorn on the way out of school? A snack alone will not ruin the whole week's meals. Think about it. These situations teach your child that it is important to be malleable in life and yet will create good memories for you!

7. Play Together

This is also easy, a delight, and one of the activities kids love most about their parents. Joking with paint, building blocks or taking that lying afternoon tea make interaction easier. Forget the mess for a few hours and let the more spontaneous and creative side of your child flow. After all, experimenting is essential for child development, and he will know that you made sure to create that kind of opportunity!

8. Let Him Help At Home

As long as activities are safe, there are only benefits in letting your child participate in household chores. Give him a piece of cloth and see how he enjoys dusting furniture or toys. Another idea is to get help to spread the sheets on the bed, store clothes in the drawers, dry plastic jars. In addition to improving motor coordination, these activities enable the child to develop a sense of responsibility and cooperation, to feel important and even more part of the family.

9. Pay Attention To The Subtleties

Learning to recognize the signs your child gives through gestures and body expressions, especially when he does not yet master speech, is a skill that strengthens the relationship. To become a master in this art, there is only one way: to pay attention. Something that seems obvious, but that can be left in a rush. So, soon you will begin to understand that that sly cry is synonymous with tiredness, what are the foods he likes best and when it is time to take a nap. And he will feel secure knowing that you understand his desires.

10. Take Photos, Make Videos...

Take a few minutes (OK, you can last for hours, get ready!) to see your child's photo albums and yours. He will love to see himself when he was little, to know what he did next to his parents, what he already said, he did ... And show his memories too. Then enjoy making funny selfies and videos (with those filters that kids love) and save them for new memories opportunities like that in the future.

11. Fill Him With Kisses And Hugs

Ah ... the best part, no? Showing affection physically is one of the most natural ways to maintain a close relationship - not to mention that touch stimulates nerve endings in the skin that promote well-being. Since you die of wanting to grab your child every time you see those cheeks even, do not hold back! Now, if he does not like hugging and kissing, that's okay. Find other ways to connect by touch, such as combing hair, moisturizer, walking hand in hand, doing a delicious massage on his feet ... And do not forget: being together is all that really matters.

Chapter 9: Toddlers: Communicating

The desire for independence: In order to become a responsible adult, your child must, as it were, move slowly from the passenger seat to the driver's seat and learn to drive the tortuous paths of life.

For children, everything is black or white For example, for a child, the concept of justice is simple: 'Mama broke a cookie and gave half to me, half to my brother.' In this case, justice comes down to a mathematical formula. Abstract thinking helps your child draw his or her own conclusions about complex issues. But this has a downside: his conclusions may be contrary to yours.

What You Can Do

Have relaxed conversations. Enjoy the moments when your child is more comfortable to talk. Be brief. You do not need to give a long sermon to every problem. Say what needs to be said and stop there. This may take effect later. When your child is alone, he will be able to think better about what you said. Give him a chance to do it.

Listen and be flexible. To get a full picture of the problem, listen carefully - without interrupting. When you say something, be reasonable. If you stick to the rules too much, your child will be tempted to look for loopholes. That's where the children begin to lead a double life. They tell parents what parents want to hear, but they do what they like when they are away from them.

Whenever possible, give guidance instead of orders. Your child's ability to think abstractly is like a muscle that needs to be exercised. So when he has to make a decision, do not do the "exercise" for him. When discussing the problem, let it suggest some solutions. Then say something like, "Now that you have given some options think of them for a day or two. Then we can talk about which one you prefer and why".

Starting from the point that parents are the best friends of children and they just want to see their happiness and satisfaction, why not be the best medium of information for them? And be able to help them?

There are many factors that cause a lack of intimacy between parents and their children, making it difficult for the family to communicate:

- Lack of meetings during meals
- Parents work late and hardly see their children
- At weekends, kids prefer television, video games or the internet than sit down for a family conversation

- When they are with their parents, the children do not expose their problems because they feel ashamed, the contact is so little that sometimes it is better to talk with a friend in the school with whom they live every day and for a certain time, than to talk with the father and mother who only finds the night and so little.

It's hard to really communicate with someone you do not know well. Do you know your child? Children need to feel that adults trust them. Many, given the opportunity, will be worthy of the trust deposited in them. And it is very good for parents to be able to speak openly and honestly about their own youth, as they did then. It shows off a high degree of confidence. Young people who can communicate with their parents are much happier and more confident. Sincere communication is the number one priority for young people. Efficient communication is based on:

- Having mutual trust.
- Show frankness and honesty.
- Be able to forgive and go forward.
- Respect privacy.
- Avoid joking and scorn.
- Maintain good humor and willingness to make real compliments
- Leave there the usual problems.
- Be able to listen and then talk.

- Move away and choose a better time when you are angry.
- Do not make accusations.

Showing interest in the children's lives is proving that parents care about them. Do you know the answers to these questions?

What is the name of your child's best friends? Have you been introduced to them yet? Do you know where they live? What kind of book, movie, and sport does your child enjoy? What is his team? What kind of music does he like? Do you know if you have any special subject, any area or hobby your child is interested in? If he practices a sport, do you know what position he plays on the team? When was the last time you went to see him play?

It is extremely important to fraternal friendship. Children need their parents more than ever, the world each day is complicated in a frightening way, several problems afflict young people, and that is why the family needs to see the lack of communication and a more intimate relationship. All major modern things, such as TV, the Internet, and advertising, contributed to the family changing their habits, greatly facilitating the lives of individuals. The truth is that there is a lack of interest of the parents in the universe of the children and vice-versa, but this has a solution, it is enough to want and to be involved.

Children with more access to language can hear up to 30 million more words by age 4 than children in unfavorable situations. How does access to language affect the development and learning of infants and toddlers? US pediatric surgeon Dana Suskind went on to investigate this issue by operating hearing-impaired babies.

She realized that among babies who received cochlear implants (deaf implants), those who best developed the ability to communicate were those who lived in homes where there were more dialogue, more interaction and more variety of vocabulary.

Their perceptions were reinforced by a 1995 study that had identified that children with less access to language (many of whom were in poverty) were able to hear 30 million fewer words accumulated up to four years of age compared to others in poorer situations favorable - and the latter were more prepared upon entering school, had richer vocabulary, more fluency in reading, and, consequently, achieved higher grades.

Since a large part of the brain growth is completed at the age of four, "children who dropped out front (in terms of language) were still ahead, those who started with lags were left behind," the study said. 'Despacito' does not leave your head? Science explains the success of the music-gum 'Children are living like rats': the plight of Mosul survivors after the expulsion of the Islamic State. To reduce these language differences in children from needy families, Suskind created in Chicago, USA , the Thirty Million Words Initiative, a program that, since motherhood and in pediatric visits, teaches parents about the importance of talking and interacting with babies from their first day of life, to stimulate the construction of new neural connections in the small brain that forms.

One of the specialist's suggestions is to tune into what your child is doing and take advantage of this to talk. The program has now been expanded to other areas of the United States, and Suskind - who is also a professor at the University of Chicago - wrote a book based on the experience: Thirty Million Words - Building a Child's Brain (Thirty Million Words - Building the Free Child Brain).

In an interview with BBC Brazil, she teaches ideas on how to use the language productively to stimulate the child's brain, which I also agree with strongly.

1. To Have Your Child As A 'Conversation Partner'

One of the first lessons of the Thirty Million Words is something intuitive for parents: to react to the sounds, looks, and gestures of the baby from birth, in a natural and integrated way to everyday life.

"If you are changing his diaper or taking a bus, explain this to the baby. It is an opportunity to enrich his vocabulary and show the relationship between a particular sound and the act to which it belongs."

Suskind cites research that shows that going beyond basic conversation - "come here," "put on your shoes," "eat your food," is a crucial point in developing children's language.

This is what she calls "extra talk," that is, dialogue with the child and the environment around her and stimulate the conversations: "what a big tree!"; "Who is the boy with the dirty diaper?"; "What is the taste of this food?"; "What do you think happened to the character in that book?"

The quantity of words is only part of the equation. The quality of the conversation is important - the richness of the vocabulary, the comings and goings of the conversation, the way you speak.

It is important to see your baby as a partner in conversations from the very first day of life.

2. Helping To Develop Mathematical Skills

Parents can help develop children's spatial sense and mathematical skills simply by talking about it.

If you use mathematical and spatial concepts - for example, counting your toes and hands, comparing the size of a triangle, using words that refer to the different shapes of objects - it will help prepare children to learn math.

A University of Chicago study asked four-year-olds to pick up punch cards drawn on them to correspond to a number (for example: when you hear the number five, pick up the card with five points drawn). And he discovered that children who had been exposed to more mathematical vocabulary and spatial notions were able to make more correct correspondences.

Moreover, Suskind argues, it is precisely in "mathematical conversations" that an important gender disparity occurs. A study of middle and upper-middle-class mothers showed that daughters as young as two heard half the mathematical conversations of their children. This may alienate girls from fields that may interest them ... Girls who hear that math is 'not their forte' often do not do well in math."

3. Speak Positively, But Praise The Effort More Than The Child

According to Suskind, children in needy families can hear more than double negative comments - "you're spoiled"; "you're wrong" - for an hour than children in families in a better socioeconomic situation.

They also hear less praise. And since these children tend to listen to fewer words in general, these negative expressions end up having a greater weight in their cognitive development. What will it be like repeatedly to hear that you never do anything right? It's a difficult child environment to overcome. The difference between prohibition words ('do not do it,' 'stop') and encouragement ('very well') is great. It causes stress in the brain to hear them repeatedly. It is important to try to change orders for a more productive conversation.

But if negative and prohibitive language can be a barrier to development and learning, is the answer always to praise - and constantly say that your child is incredible and intelligent?

There has been researching, showing that this kind of praise can, rather than empower future adults, only leave them passive and dependent on the opinion of others. What we are looking for is not the eyes facing themselves, happy with self-satisfaction, but children who see a task and, no matter how challenging it may be, can almost immediately think how it can be fulfilled. It's what parents want: adults stable, constructive, motivated.

The way to do this, according to the studies analyzed by Suskind, is to recognize and praise not only the child, but the effort and commitment of it in their daily activities, the use of other words, instead of just saying "you're too smart" to a girl who turned a difficult puzzle, go further: "I saw you struggled to finish and succeeded. Very well! "

Suskind suggests looking for day-to-day moments when the child has stood out. The child is still learning what it is to behave well. Pointing these moments to her reinforces the idea of what that means.

4. Stimulate Autonomy Rather Than Just Obedience

Suskind quotes two sentences that can be said to a child in the same context:

"Now store your toys."

"What should we do with toys after we've finished playing?"

"The first sentence is an order that must be fulfilled without questioned. The second sentence, however, supports the autonomy of the child. One-year-old babies whose mothers are quietly suggesting, rather than ordering, behavioral rules have gained executive function and self-regulation by the age of four "- which are our ability to stay focused on a problem instead of react explosively and violently. Parents who use the pressure and the authority to restrict the child's behavior can get obedience in the short term, but in the long, are creating conditions for low self-regulation (the child).

The least efficient method of constructing brain connections because it is the most efficient method of constructing brain connections require no or little language response. It may be more efficient, instead of just saying" put on your shoes, "explaining what is behind the request and the relationship between cause and effect of things:" It's time to go to school. glue, so it's good to put your shoes on to keep your feet dry and warm. Please go get them."

5. Tune In To The Child - And Indulge In The" Baby Voice"

Suskind recommends paying attention to what is arousing the child's interest - a joke, an object - and turn it around on the topic of conversation. Another example: The father or mother, with the best of intentions, sits on the floor next to the child with a children's book in their hands. But the child does not pay attention and continues to play with his toy, snobbery the adult. The parent gives direct and short orders like "sit," "stay quiet," and "do not do it." Now, these are the least efficient method of building brain connections because they require little or no language response.

How about instead of imposing the reading of the book, entering into the child's play and talking about it? Parents learn to become aware of what their children are doing and become part of it, helping to develop practiced ability the play and, through verbal interaction, the child's brain. Tuning in also involves, according to her, to take every opportunity to read and sing with the child - or even speak with that infantile voice that many of us use with babies.

"That sung voice is a rich nutrient for the baby's brain because it helps him understand the sounds of words," explains Suskind. Here's one more warning: An easy way to lose that harmony with children and infants is to be distracted by the cell phone during the game. Smartphones are taking the place of personal interaction with infants and children. It is only when the child is the primary focus of parents that attention is needed for optimal brain development.

Chapter 10: Family Routines

How Can Routine Help Your Child?

We know that in practice, it is not easy to establish a routine in the lives of children, especially with the rush of everyday life, irregular hours, and lack of time. However, it is very important that the family adopt some habits and rules in the daily life of the little ones. A routine for children, from an early age, helps them to grow more confident and independent. Knowing what will happen during the day, and repeating these events creates a healthy environment, making the children feel comfortable and safe.

Little ones like to know what will happen during their day. Knowing that, after a nap, is the snack or that, before bed, is the story, provides a sense of security. This makes the little ones feel less anxious. Over time, the routine can even cause your baby to develop certain mania, such as sleeping with the same blanket or just eating certain foods. It is the way they have to feel in control, in this world still so foreign to them.

Benefits for Dads and Moms

For parents, pre-established routines also bring many benefits. First, because they feel more secure, the little ones tend to accept the farewell moments better. For example, the time to leave the playground or say goodbye when parents go to work does not become so difficult because they understand that they will return. Thus, from an early age, the little ones will understand and assimilate the schedules and rules of everyday life. When they grow up, they become children and adolescents with a greater sense of organization and responsibility, being able to establish study and bonding schedules, such as helping the family in household activities. In addition, routines also help organize the life of parents. Having established schedules for meals, naps, showers, and games, makes the whole family organize better and have more time to enjoy the moments together.

Know How To Be Flexible

It is important to remember that the excess is never good and therefore not worth turning the house into a barracks! You have to know the time to be flexible so that the routine does not become something negative. On weekends, for example, you are allowed to sleep a few more hours or have lunch later. The important thing is to set schedules and create healthy habits that make the environment more organized and comfortable for everyone!

Bedtime

Bedtime is the first routine idea of the little ones, and they need to know the difference between day and night. Naps during the day should always be in a clear environment, without disturbing noises or changing the routine of the house.

For night sleep parents need to perform "sleep hygiene" as a ritual. It can be a relaxing bath, followed by a story. The room should be dimly lit and free of noise.

Time To Feed

It is healthy to have family meals, all seated at the table and tasting varied foods. Take the opportunity to talk and realize that your little one is growing. You can also enjoy setting up a new menu for the following week.

Establish Schedules

It is important that children have schedules to wake up, carry out activities, play, and sleep. Following the schedule makes the child get used to it and establishes a routine. You can assemble for your little one a timesheet with drawings, showing what will be the order of your day, this will bring more security to him.

Organized Spaces

Having an organized environment will help the little ones. For this to happen, it is very important that they know that:

- After playing, they should store their toys
- Used clothes should be placed in the basket

From an early age, the little ones can and should help with the housework, after all, they are also part of the house!

What Is The Importance Of Routine For The Child?

Routine exerts a fundamental influence on child development. Among other factors, it teaches the child to live with family and even community reality (neighborhood, school, etc.), in addition to contributing to the strengthening of autonomy. But only 15% of the population considers it important that the child up to 3 years of age have a routine (food, bath, hours to watch television, etc.).

What Exactly Is Routine?

Value the role of routine in early childhood, always respecting diversity. Each family has its own way of working. In communication, reinforce that children should have sleep, food, hygiene, and playtime and that this is good for their development.

What Are The Benefits Of Routine For The Child?

The establishment of the routine is very important for the child and for his adult life. The adult you will be, depends on your experience as a child. Childhood is when you establish a strong sense of self and routine reinforces a positive self-image. In this sense, the benefits of the routine can be summarized as: In order for the child to feel safe, he has to acquire positive and healthy habits from the beginning. Children do not know the order of things when they are born, and so it is adults who must teach them to organize their lives through schedules associated with routines, that is, through activities they must do every day in the same way.

The repetition of rituals helps the child to assimilate an inner scheme that makes the world a predictable and therefore safe place.

Food, sleep, and hygiene are the first habits that children have to learn. The daily routine is for children what the walls are for the home; it gives them limits and dimensions of life. The routine gives a sense of security. The established routine gives a sense of order from which freedom is born.

What Do Habits And Routines For Children Mean?

The routine is a personal custom established by your coexistence and does not allow modification, that is, it is inflexible, safeguarded some very specific situations that are beyond our control, such as unforeseen events. The habit is a stable mechanism that creates skills and can be used in a variety of situations, such as putting on seat belts. Habits are customs, attitudes, behaviors, or behaviors that imply learning. The well-used and used habit allows us to face everyday events.

Habits and routines contribute to constancy and regularity, important mechanisms, and therefore are fundamental for both family and school life.

What Are The Consequences Of Lack Of Routine For The Child?

Not having a basic routine brings behavioral problems that can be considered inconvenient by an inexperienced professional; in school, the child may present difficulties that are often also perceived as Learning Disorders. In addition, the child becomes disorganized, giving more work than usual. The construction of the personality can also be affected since the routine has limits and rules necessary and fundamental for the construction of the character of the person. Children crave control, just as adults do. Without a routine, they may feel that they have none, and this can result in anxiety and tantrums.

How Can We Establish A Healthy Routine For Children?

First of all, be aware of what each child can do at the age they are. Give autonomy forever. Do not raise your children as if they were princes or princesses. They need to learn early on that they are ordinary people just like any other. Time to sleep, wake up, play.

Create habits and rules: brush your teeth after meals, do the chores first, and play later.

Teach them to organize their own objects and toys.

Always speak the truth so that the child does not learn to lie at home.

At mealtimes and on homework, the TV, tablet, and mobile phone should be out of the reach of the child so as not to compete with what needs to be done.

Teach your children that you, parents, are the people of authority at home! Children do not tell their parents what to do but can instead share their opinions on a subject. Be in charge, but don't forget to be flexible and remember that you are growing tiny adults. You must be the people of affective and authoritative reference to your children. Do not delegate to others the education and rearing of your children. The real presence of the parents is fundamental to the development of the child. Stay tuned to the way they talk, how they dress, how they behave. Your children observe your ways of being and adopt your habits as their own. Sometimes the behavioral problem that the child presents originates from the home itself.

Follow the evolution of your children in school, and in the face of difficulties, seek help as soon as possible. Take care of your children's self-esteem! Do not call them by nicknames and/or negative words. This affects the self-esteem and emotional growth of your children. Set small tasks so that the children also contribute to the proper functioning of the house.

And remember, a well-educated child from an early age will be a responsible and happy adult in the future!

Making Family – Make Children Confident!

What is breakfast like at your house? So much rush that your son can only finish the sandwich inside the car? And at dinner is everyone so tired that all you can do is throw yourself on the couch and eat some pasta? Okay, we know routine is crazy now, but - maybe - it's time to rethink some habits.

A survey of 34,000 children and adolescents from the Literacy Trust, an English institution dedicated to literacy and reading encouragement, concluded that talking during meals helps raise more confident children. To reach this result, the children responded as it was the time of the meals in their homes and some questions that indirectly evaluated their social and communicative abilities.

The survey found that 87 percent of the children sat with their families during the meal, but one in four did not talk to their parents or siblings. Among those who always ate with their parents and talked during meals, 75% said they feel comfortable to participate in classroom discussions. Among those who did not talk, that number dropped to 57%. When asked how they felt about talking in front of friends in the class, in the first group, 62% said they felt good compared to 47% in the second. Through these parameters, those in charge of the research concluded that talking during meals is a great tool for children and parents.

Research shows the importance of family communication. A table is a place that favors this union because people need to be seated if they look in the eye, and the dialogue happens. But these exchanges should not happen only in those moments.

For families living in large urban centers, it is difficult to demand that they make the three meals together. The tip is to try to reserve at least one of them to sit down and eat calmly. If a parent has no time to get home, try to organize the routine in the morning for family coffee. If the nights are quieter, eat together for dinner. The most important thing is that the meal is well-made, and you have time to talk. Knowing how the day was, what's new at school, if he's enjoying swimming lessons, if he's spoken to his grandmother. The main thing is interaction and that parents show interest in their children's lives.

If your family's routine is too rushed or if your children are still small and make meals much earlier than the rest of the house, do not despair. Although the table is a strong symbol of family unity, you can reinvent the moments of coexistence. Keeping this dialogue while you are stuck in traffic with the kids in the car, telling bedtime stories and enjoying every weekend minute are viable alternatives for busy families.

Another important tip: do not let the technology stay between you. At mealtime, turn off the television. Check emails on your smartphone? Forget. Leave to use these accessories when alone.

What Does The Family Meal Do For You?

According to nutritionist Marisa Resende Coutinho, from São Camilo Hospital (SP), family meals are fundamental for the formation of food habits. The younger children are still learning to eat. We need to put food on the table, make them taste, and see what they're eating.

In addition, watching what parents are eating stimulates the child's curiosity. Parents are a great example in relation to food. It's no good if you want your child to eat carrots if he's never seen you do it. The same goes for foods that you do not want to present to your child: if the idea is to delay soda intake, for example, avoid taking that tin in front of the children - they are sure to ask you to try it!

From 6 months on, it's time to introduce solid foods into your child's diet. At about 10 months, your child is already able to sit, so you can stay in the high chair by the table. If it is already adapted to the solids, there is no problem in offering the same food as the parents, provided it is prepared with a little seasoning. Another difference is that the food should cook a bit more to become softer and facilitate the ingestion.

Chapter 11: Rules And Consequences

Everything that is little has grace, but when the little one realizes that he has his own wills, grace can turn into disgrace! We speak, of course, of the phases of tantrums, spoiled, and uncontrollable children who do not give us rest. Like any human being, kids also need basic rules to be able to explore and avenge in their little world ... without leaving their parents on the verge of a fit of nerves.

The Importance of Rules and Limits

The American pediatrician Berry Brazelton says that "for children to grow well, they need only love and limits" - love is fundamental to growing with confidence and self-esteem; limits are crucial for the child to learn self-control so that he can live in a family and in society. That is, with respect to the rules of behavior at home (and out of it!) Is really "small that twists the cucumber." Education starts at home, and you do not have to feel guilty for being too strict - children become balanced adults because they lived by rules and limits, not the other way around.

Few And Good

Child behavior studies show that children respond very well to rules, provided they are simple and limited in quantity. Once the child is old enough to see what is right and wrong, make the rules that are appropriate to their age, clearly and one at a time, so as not to confuse them. It is better to memorize fewer than none. Without losing authority or making many concessions, try to maintain some flexibility: for example, when explaining to the child this or that situation, give them three possible scenarios, asking them to give their opinion as to which way to go. In addition to engaging and fostering their independence, it makes limit enforcement less rigid and less "heavy," with "negotiation" being the easiest way for kids to learn to respect the rules. Of course, establishing and imposing limits on your little angels will sometimes cost you (it's a normal feeling), it will not be easy, and it will take time. But patience, love, and joint learning will give precious help.

How To Set Rules

When you want to implement a rule, talk to your child calmly, explaining what you want as clearly as possible, asking you several times if you have questions. Explain to him the consequences of non-compliance with the rules. The "punishments" should be very clear and executable, that is, do not say that you will deprive you of watching television for a week if you know that you will never have the courage to do so. Give the child some freedom in complying with the rules, that is, if he knows that at 9:00 pm he has clean up the toys, brush his teeth and get to bed, let him choose what he wants to do first. Rules can also be fun!

I Was Wrong!

If the child "threatens" does not comply with one of the rules, give him a 5-minute warning, speaking calmly but seriously and remind him of the consequences. After checking that the rule has not been fulfilled or has been partially fulfilled, ask why the child did not do it, explain how you do it (in case you had any difficulty) or help him finish the task, saying that for the next it will be able to do it alone. The easiest way for a child to try to get out of complying with their rules is to make a tantrum. However, adults should never give in to children's tantrums. If you get to the point where punishment is necessary, do not hesitate to stick to it, that is, do not change your mind, do not change the "promised" punishment - otherwise you may get the idea that the consequences are not real and does or does not enforce the rules.

You Did Well!

Do not focus too much on bad behavior and try to give equal attention to good behavior. When children put their books away or wash their hands without anyone telling you anything, praise and pamper them - there is nothing that children enjoy more than being the target of parental attention (for a good reason!), so it is natural that they continue to behave well, just to continue to draw their attention. When the child behaves and asks for something calmly and politely, consider making him feel comfortable.

Some of the best rules you can establish for children to behave well:

Establishing rules for children is fundamental to early childhood education because it is through them that it is possible to teach limits and develop the capacity to live in society. However, it is not enough just to determine what your child can and cannot do: you need to explain why these standards exist and are so important.

Many parents believe that children cannot assimilate this kind of information, but that is a mistake. Despite their young age, children are able to absorb and understand a lot of information. Of course, they do not have the same degree of understanding as adults, but they can already understand some important aspects of rules and norms.

Parents need not only cherish the physical and mental health of their children but also provide a quality education so that they can live in society, respecting the limits of the child and understanding how the mechanisms work. To help you make your child behave, we have mentioned some rules for children that all parents must put into practice.

Always greet and say goodbye when in any setting

No matter if the child is in the home, at school, or anywhere else, she needs to say hello and say goodbye to the people who are present in the environment in which he finds himself. That's a way for him always to tell us when he's here or when he's leaving. More than that: this is a basic etiquette standard for any occasion.

Tidying Up Everything He Has Disrupted, Or Parents Ask For

This is perhaps one of the rules for older children to teach the child. Your child needs to be aware that everything he or she takes off must be replaced immediately after use. This is true for toys, books, clothes, etc. But it's not just what the child has messed with. He needs to be aware that the family environment is a space of shared coexistence, so everyone needs to help.

Laying the table, taking things to the sink, helping folding clothes, are little organizing activities that will make all the difference in her future.

Always Use "Please" When You Ask For Something

This word, "please," may seem like just details, but it makes all the difference in kindergarten. With it, the child understands that it is necessary to ask for things with education, to be attended to (if possible), and not just imposing their will.

This is one of the rules for children that needs to be constantly demonstrated by parents. If the child sees the mother or father demanding things without asking please, of course, she will imitate them. So it's up to the parents to set the example accordingly.

Apologizing

Knowing how to make a mistake is another fundamental item for early childhood education, as this will directly interfere with the child's personality in the future. A child who does not assume that he has done the wrong thing will become an inconsequential adult, who will have no remorse for wrongdoings, even if they harm others.

A good way to encourage and teach your child to apologize is to decrease your punishment. If he makes a mistake and promises that he will no longer commit (or will only try to avoid) the punishment should be less. But he needs attention so that he does not end up apologizing just for not being punished.

No Swearing

This is also one of the rules for children that many parents have difficulty teaching to children. This is often because they themselves cannot control vocabulary around children, or because they end up being exposed to such words in other settings, such as at school or at family events, for example.

In order for children to not speak profanity, the first step is for parents to cut off this kind of language from day to day. Remember: you are the mirror of your child. If this type of verbiage is used in other settings such as a family party, get close to relatives and explain that you do not want them to use these words so that the child is not influenced.

Not Playing With Food Or Grumbling At The Table

This is a common household problem. The child seems just to want to play, or if he does not like something, he grumbles how much he hates a certain type of food. In those hours, it takes patience. Sit down with your child and explain why he should be polite to the table, not complaining about the food. If he does not like something, like vegetables (which is very common), explain how important they are to his health, to growing. Do all this without forgetting, of course, to lead by example, behaving well at the table and having a healthy diet.

Do Not Waste

Sustainability is also a subject that must be present when it comes to teaching rules for children. They need to learn that every little thing, whether it's a lighted light or a dripping faucet, makes all the difference for the protection of the environment.

Teach the child never to waste things. When leaving an environment, always turn off the light, close the taps well, do not put on the dish what he will not be able to eat, among other things. In this way, it will create environmental awareness from an early age.

Always Pay Attention When Someone Is Talking To You And Talk Politely

The last of the rules for children fundamental to early childhood education is that the child is always educated. This should be present, whether in the way of talking to other adults or children or listening to someone talking to them. This teaching will interfere with her whole life. For the child to learn this, obviously parents need to set an example. If the child wants to tell you something, do not ignore it or pretend to listen. Give the attention he needs. The same goes for talking to him: be polite and keep the tone appropriate for the conversation.

What Mistakes To Avoid So Rules For Children Work

Many parents complain that they try to teach rules for children, but it seems that they do not change anything in the way they are. Probably this is because you, as a parent, are committing one of the following errors:

- Do not impose limits of truth, just speak the rules to children out of mouth
- Teach one thing, but do another
- Do not remember every day how important these standards are
- Just introduce the rules for children without explaining why they exist.

Those are just a few mistakes. By avoiding them, you will find it much easier to educate your child. It is these vices that many adults have that end up harming the child's learning, causing it to repeat the same bad habits of the parents. When teaching rules for children, always keep in mind that this is a continuous and joint work. This means that it needs to happen on a daily basis and that parents also need to show that they are following the same standards so that the child understands that it is valid for all.

Educating children is a complicated task. It requires creativity, authority, persistence, determination ... As each child acts in a way, some parents are more likely to impose limits than others. But it's obvious that they all need to set rules for the little ones to respect. Punishment? Spanking? Conversation?

Each one has his way of acting, which can please others or not. But there are some basic tips that all parents (and grandparents, uncles ...) can follow and that help in the education of a child. However, this is not a cake recipe. Each family needs to fit their reality and the reality of their child. It does not cost a try.

1 - Limit For The Children, Not For The Parents

You establish a rule and impose it for your child. However, it requires that you also follow it. This is very common in the education process, but it cannot always be applied. The limits are for the children, not for the parents. It is the children who are being educated, not their parents. It's always good to keep that in mind.

It is obvious that parents need to be the example; this is very important for the fixation of learning. But it is essential to know that this part of each adult is not an obligation, nor is it allowed for the little ones to dictate similar rules and apply them. If this is happening in your home, you better cut it.

2 - Consequences Of Acts Need To Be Fulfilled

It is almost obvious that if you spoke, they must comply. Therefore, if you have established a rule and said what would be the consequence if the limit was broken, you should put it into practice. It is logical, and in this way, the child will know that you are not speaking for speaking and will respect what you have established without questioning.

However, just as a consequence cannot be "let go," they should not last for long, months, for example, or be permanent. The child needs to be aware of why he was punished. If the punishment is for an indeterminate time, it will come an hour that she will no longer know the reason and will feel wronged.

3 - Rules For Young Children

Many parents are afraid to set rules and limits for small children, but to begin with, this process of education as soon as possible allows children to respect parents at the exact moment of each stage of their life. And believe me, even the young at a very young age already understand what you mean.

Start by imposing rules such as the right time to eat, take a shower, to go to bed. Do everything exactly the same way, every day. Surely you will have fewer problems when you need to send your children to school or do your homework, for example, because they will know you are not kidding.

4 - No Repetitions

You established the rule and applied it. He explained the acts and consequences to his son and made him understand everything right. All right. Now, let the child watch over and take care of one's behavior. Nothing of repeating the same rule at all times, tiring the child and even himself. This will often end up making your child want to see what happens if she breaks that rule so fixed. And if he does, go back to tip 2 of that list: apply the consequence firmly. So, you will be showing to the child that everything he said is valid and that you give the final word.

5 - Limit Age For The Rules

Some parents will ask themselves: should I set limits until my child is at what age? This is relative, and each family has its own culture; each child has his way of acting. But definitely, there is no age limit to stop applying the rules. This should happen as long as the children depend on their parents. From babies to adulthood, if they live under your roof, your kids need you in some way. So rules need to be put in place for a good coexistence, without them overriding your authority. When they are independent and self-reliant, they will set the rules of their own home.

6 - Establishing The Rules

You do not have to create a rule, establish it, but when you apply it, end up seeing that it is a failure. So it is very important to see and revise the limits as often as necessary so that when it comes to putting them into practice, you can show the children exactly what they did and what rules they broke.

Faulty rules are dangerous because children always end up finding a way to circumvent what you have set up, and then you will not have to argue. It is good for parents to make the rules together, even if they are separate. Thus, the child will know that what is worth in one's house is also worth in the house of the other.

7 - Parent Involvement

Depending on the age of your child, he or she may not have discernment of what is right and wrong, and it is up to you to set boundaries. However, from the age of the child to adolescence, they know exactly what they do, what is good or bad, what is according to their demands or not, anyway. Therefore, it may be interesting that they participate in the definition of rules and limits. What happens if they do this or that, what their opinion about some acts, what they think about what you think is wrong, among other things. However, make it clear that it is you who gives the final word and determines the rule in your home.

8 - Be Persistent

Be consistent and consistent in rules. If you break the limits yourself, you end up losing credibility with your children. It seems obvious that they will think, "If he himself could not keep what he said, what can he say about me?" The firm wrist is the watchword for a good education. Create rules consistently so that it fits into the family's everyday life and that everyone living under one roof can collaborate with the child's education. Each family has its reality, and it is very important that the boundaries fit perfectly so that you also do not make your child have a justification for failure.

9 - Visits To Children

If you establish a rule for your child, it will also apply to friends who visit them inside your home. And you should make sure the child or teen explains the rules to other people so that the whole family is not misunderstood, and everyone can live together harmoniously.

Two examples: If you do not want your children to play on the couch, they should tell their friends that it is forbidden in your home. Or if you do not allow your teen to consume alcohol inside your home, you need to make sure their friends know that the party at your house will not have anything of the kind.

10 - In And Out Of Home

Before leaving home, remind your children that the same rules you apply there, are also valid for when they are out. Make it clear that if a boundary break occurs when you are in someone's home, the consequences will apply when they arrive, with no chance of escape. And, if necessary, do so. Try to talk to the child's grandparents, so they do not allow things you do not like, like eating in front of the TV, for example. If something like this happens, remind your children that it happened only once because the grandparents left, but it will not happen again, not here or at your house.

Establishing rules, imposing limits, and applying consequences to children, especially when they are small, can be tricky and even painful for parents. But this will result in responsible adults who know how to respect the world in which they live. A service that parents provide their children with a medium and long-term result.

Conclusion

Understanding the behavior of your toddler may not be the easiest thing to do, however, with a little effort and the right guidance you will be able to raise your kid in a way you will be proud of. Parenting is not something you learn to master overnight, it's an ongoing process, and the more time you invest in getting it right, the more obstacles you'll face! That's not a bad thing. It is an indication you are eager to learn more and improve as a parent.

This book is crafted for you to address some of the most common problems you will face as a parent and help you to deal with it more effectively.

While we have covered a lot of information regarding children and toddlers and their behavior, you need to remember that every child is different and what works like a charm for one kid may prove to be ineffective for your kid. That doesn't mean these techniques aren't helpful. It just means you need to customize the technique a little to benefit your child. As a parent, you know your kid better than anyone else. With the information in this book and your expertise, you should be able to come up with a plan that works well for you and your child!

Do let us know how this book helped you by leaving a review. This will encourage eager parents to make the right purchase.
Happy Parenting!

www.ingramcontent.com/pod-product-compliance
Lightning Source LLC
Chambersburg PA
CBHW020354080526
44584CB00014B/1010